Complementary, Alternative Methods and Supplementary Medicine

Other World Scientific Titles by the Author

The Angiology Bible
by G Belcaro
ISBN: 978-1-78634-569-1

Noninvasive Investigations in Vascular Disease
by G Belcaro and A N Nicolaides
ISBN: 978-1-86094-213-6

Once We Were Hunters: A Study of the Evolution of Vascular Disease
by G Belcaro
ISBN: 978-1-86094-262-4 (pbk)

Pharma-Standard Supplements: Clinical Use
by G Belcaro
ISBN: 978-1-78326-933-4
ISBN: 978-1-78326-934-1 (pbk)

The Venous Clinic: Diagnosis, Prevention, Investigations, Conservative and Medical Treatment, Sclerotherapy and Surgery
by G Belcaro, A N Nicolaides and G Stansby
ISBN: 978-1-86094-051-4

Complementary, Alternative Methods and Supplementary Medicine

Giovanni Vincent Belcaro
Irvine[3] Vascular Lab, Ch-Pe University, Italy

Supervised by Dr. Maria Rosaria Cesarone

World Scientific
NEW JERSEY • LONDON • SINGAPORE • BEIJING • SHANGHAI • HONG KONG • TAIPEI • CHENNAI • TOKYO

Published by

World Scientific Publishing Europe Ltd.

57 Shelton Street, Covent Garden, London WC2H 9HE

Head office: 5 Toh Tuck Link, Singapore 596224

USA office: 27 Warren Street, Suite 401-402, Hackensack, NJ 07601

Library of Congress Cataloging-in-Publication Data
Names: Belcaro, Giovanni Vincent, author.
Title: Complementary, alternative methods and supplementary medicine / by
Giovanni Vincent Belcaro (Irvine[3] Vascular Lab, Ch-Pe University, Italy).
Description: New Jersey : World Scientific, 2018.
Identifiers: LCCN 2018020242 | ISBN 9781786345660 (hc : alk. paper)
Subjects: | MESH: Complementary Therapies | Dietary Supplements |
Phosphatidylserines--therapeutic use | Medicine, Traditional
Classification: LCC R733 | NLM WB 890 | DDC 615.8/8--dc23
LC record available at https://lccn.loc.gov/2018020242

British Library Cataloguing-in-Publication Data
A catalogue record for this book is available from the British Library.

For any available supplementary material, please visit
https://www.worldscientific.com/worldscibooks/10.1142/Q0168#t=suppl

Desk Editors: Anthony Alexander/Jennifer Brough/Shi Ying Koe

Typeset by Stallion Press
Email: enquiries@stallionpress.com

To Natalie, the everlasting inspirations

Foreword

Since mankind has had memory, health has always meant a series of things such as happiness, wealth, power and supremacy. At the same time, lack of health has also represented fear, pain, survival and death. These are just a very few answers to a simple question like "what does health mean to you?", and these are the most frequent replies. The answers may change according to latitudes and to places where people live and circumstances that are occurring at that moment. The meaning of health also changes itself according to historical events and is different if in peaceful times rather than in war times.

Good health means wellness, and this also leads to the concepts such as growing a family, improving beauty and making money. At the same time, health conditions can change professional conditions, jobs, skills and other most challenging situations. Health-influencing herbs, drugs and even mind-conditioning treatments are capable of changing strength, temper, resistance and will of a person.

The figure of the "wealth man" is old as mankind's memory goes back, but if we are willing to observe nature and its environs, we can see and distinguish a healthy animal from a sick one, one that perhaps has wounds and consequently is starving or cannot defend himself from other perils.

From here, it is easy to understand the idea that a healthy community can help the sick one, while a lonely element is by itself and also weaker when unhealthy. For this reason, the "health man" has always distinguished himself, being both powerful and feared by the community. With time, the man that actually *cured the disease* also began teaching *why and how to do the job* gaining the definition of *doctor* (from the latin *docere*). Of course being a doctor in China was, and maybe still is, different than being one in Africa or in the Andes, but the searched result always is the same: wellness with health. Still, in every part of the world, the word "doctor" means the same thing even if the methods may change and above all the cures may vary, sometimes even very much because of local traditions.

At present, medical drugs with their use and evolution have achieved global distribution and prescription patterns. Diseases and treatments are now quite comparable in different nations. In other words, there is also globalization in diseases and in some remedies.

Nevertheless, in these most recent years, we are witnessing a continuous evolution of *how* to deal with and treat diseases. People are searching for alternative cures and methods, and more often, these remedies are searched for amongst nonqualified "medicine treatments". This definition is actually very generic, and so the correct one should be distinguished by "official" and "alternative and complementary". Even the so-called "official" medicine may be different dependent upon latitudes, countries and available wealth conditions.

Paradoxically, world globalization is also introducing "alternative medicine" and even "do-it-yourself". Moreover, media and the worldwide web have created a parallel world where increasingly often "real and by law" doctors are totally skipped over by parallel medicine practitioners.

Listening every day to remonstrance and criticisms towards medical doctors and general practice as a whole, the first problem is bureaucracy, which takes more of a medical doctor's time than actually doing the healing. From here, the step is quite short to frustration by patients, and thus a growing number of patients look for "alternative" cures rather than wait for doctors to take time off from administrating and to return to healing. Their health conditions are or may be dangerous, and above all, there is so much confusion amongst the "alternative" cures that some distinctions require adequate attention, and only doctors can provide this healing knowledge and attention.

This book, divided into arguments and sections and easy to read, is perhaps one of the most distinguished attempts to explain alternative and complementary medicine and should be read by both medical practitioners and by their patients. It is a clear roadmap to distinguish what to do and, above all, *what not to do*. A guide such as this book has been absolutely missing from modern libraries, and I am grateful to the authors for their work, particularly that they have made such a complex topic much more simple and palatable.

I am also grateful to Dr. Maria Rosaria Cesarone for the careful supervision and planning of this work.

Peter M. Bavera, MD
Vascular Surgeon and Diagnostician

About the Author

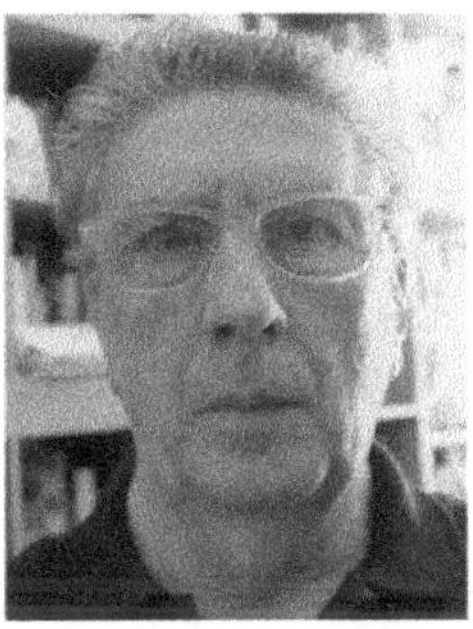

Giovanni V Belcaro is the founder of the Irvine[3] Vascular Lab, Ch-Pe University, Italy and the leader of the San Valentino Vascular Screening Project. He obtained his degree in Medicine and Surgery, then specialized in general surgery and subsequently in thoracic surgery. He obtained a PhD from the University College (St. Mary's Hospital Campus), London working with Mr. HHG Eastcott and Prof. AN Nicolaides. He has obtained the Imperial College Certificate in Vascular Surgery and Microcirculation (UCL, London). He is a fellow of the Royal Society of Medicine, London, UK, a British Council scholar and has worked at Bispebjerg Hospital, Copenhagen. He has authored 30 books and more than 500 scientific articles and original papers. He has attended 300 international meetings. Presentations include those at Westminster and at the European Parliament. He is a member of the editorial board of several international journals. He has worked and operated in different projects in several places including Africa, Philippines, Japan, China, Pakistan and Afghanistan. Among the many research projects he completed, he was the first to implant an artificial Gore-Tex venous valve and to use lymphatic transplant. His work on early atherosclerotic plaques evaluation and screening has been a significant progress in the early management of atherosclerosis.

Contents

Part 1
Complementary and Alternative Medicine

1
Introduction

Complementary and alternative medicine (CAM) is a commonly accepted term that is not completely correct from many points of view. It is probably better to indicate these nonstandard medical methods as "supportive medicine" instead of CAM. Some concepts like "well-being" — very often mentioned and an easy target for CAM — are not logical, scientific, physiological concepts. Well-being is very individual and it is not a treatable disease. Management of aging is another popular target with minimal or no scientific or clinical credibility. The transformation of doctors and qualified practitioners into undefined "healers" is always suspicious and it does not add credibility to the methods.

New Age Hippies have spread a sort of religion assisted by useless zeal. The fantastic images of Edward Hicks (*The Peaceful Kingdom* in all its approximately 80 versions) in which leopards and lambs, children and lions or wolves, colonist and natives live in peace and harmony have been virtually extended to viruses, bacteria and tumor cells in a kind of "all friends together" mentality, which leads the ignorant and uninformed to some dangerous conclusions.

Some spiritual concepts have been wildly incorporated by the post-Hippy, postindustrial, postreligious, metropolitan Indians, friend of the viruses, pseudo-Zen and followers of modified oriental-style doctrines. Wild notions have been wildly incorporated into "traditional" or "mainstream medicine". "Spiritual" concepts do not need any clinical or scientific validation or even basic physiological explanation. Yet, in medicine, "traditional" does not mean bad and it does not mean good either. It must be evaluated according to some logic. "Older" does not mean better. The context is of the essence. What was valid in a small rural village in China in a period of very limited options is quite possibly not the best option now.

Complementary medicine and alternative medicine are still fairly misleading terms, and differently accepted concepts and terms (according to cultures and social interactions), and are still not clear to many patients. Medicine is either yes or no, in or out. There is no alternative. Some *alternative–complementary healing methods* are used often without a specific diagnostic process and for conditions that are not diseases. The concept of accurate dosage appears to be alien to most of these systems. Also, medicine (mainstream or standard medicine, MSM) by law should be practiced *only* by qualified and certified professionals. However, most unconventional alternative methods are used in many situations by unqualified "healers". In some cases, professionals are not available, and so alternative or traditional local methods are used for cultural reasons as a result of a lack of mainstream standard medical facilities or for many other reasons including ideology and ignorance when there is no doctor.

According to the Merck Manual, medicine is defined as alternative when use is made of unconventional practices which have not been validated by mainstream medicine or, which do not have a defined, logical, scientific background. Complementary medicine may indicate a set of unconventional peri medical practices and systems using untested healing practices and methods that can be used in association with mainstream medicine. Integrative medicine uses all defined approaches of medicine including alternative practices in a framework that focuses on the whole person. This definition is actually quite meaningless, as good "standard" medicine — when properly applied — is already focused on the entire patient. The fact that complementary and alternative medicine are widely used is not a certification. Also, the cost to the customer of some complementary and alternative therapies may imply that these methods have a more significant value for some patients. Often patients do not tell their physicians about alternative–complementary or integrative methods and the products they use. But physicians need to evaluate potential dangers or identify possible interactions.

The use of CAM in its unidentified galaxy of practices varies from country to country; these methods may help some patients or give them consolation and the impression that some action is in progress when other methods fail, have failed or are not convincing. For these subjects, CAM is a strong temptation and often they see these practices as their only remaining solution and hope. Some points may support the use of specific CAMs (i.e., acupuncture):

- Some healing methods have been used for ages with anecdotal reports of success.
- Some physiological methods or evaluation systems have shown an activity of the healing methods.
- Some clinical studies or GCP trials have shown real efficacy.

The fact that there is no evidence or limited evidence for a specific practice is also misleading. Evidence is searched with resources and persistence (clinical trials) when there is a significant profit to be made or a patent to defend. Most methods and products in CAM are not patentable and therefore do not constitute a significant market to exploit. No profit, no evidence: simple.

Most healing methods are difficult to test and there is no incentive in showing efficacy, because somebody somewhere will always "believe" in them, proof or no proof. Most methods appear to be based on the efficacy of the healer: what he can do cannot be reproduced by others. This concept implies something like sanctity which does not belong to mainstream medicine.

Supplementary medicine (using supplements in pharmaceutical standards) is a different story. Modern products (generally of natural origin) — available in raw form for many years — can now be produced and used according to state of the art pharmaceutical standards. These may be defined as pharma-standard (PS) supplements. An original natural product (e.g., curcumin) with new methods of extraction and purification (i.e., not involving chemicals) is refined, standardized, minimized: new procedures ensure that there are no contaminants (heavy metals, pesticides) even in minimal quantities; the absorption is stable and consistent. With new procedures, its supplementary value becomes quite different from the effects derived from the use of "raw, natural" material.

Most PS supplements are "recognized as safe" (RAS) and have a safety factor much higher than many drugs that have been tested in a relatively small number of patients for a relatively small period of time. These supplements have been tested for centuries in millions of subjects and in some populations, a specific culture has grown around their use, activities, applications and anecdotes about potential dangers or interactions. Most supplementary products in the format of PS supplements can now be tested almost as drugs in specific conditions — and their results can be standardized.

Studies on interactions between PS supplements and drugs are in progress. Any contamination from poisonous substances is now out of question in high-quality PS supplements while this is not possible with "herbal" preparations or nonstandardized products. Interaction between "natural", nonstandardized products may cause important alterations in the efficacy of many therapies. All CAM therapies must be considered within context because even apparently simple methods, such as physical manipulations or acupuncture (i.e., in subjects using anticoagulants), may result in complications such as bleeding problems and hematomas. Any CAM procedure or healing proposal should be always discussed with a physician and formally approved. The *Merck Manual* has the best definitions and classifications for these procedures. The manual recognizes five types of "alternative" or peri medical methods are as follows:

- alternative "medical" systems,
- mind–body medical methods,
- biological practices,
- manipulative and body-based practices,
- energy medical methods.

2

Alternative Whole Medical Systems

Ayurveda

Ayurveda is a traditional "medical" complex and system of rules used in India for more than 4,000 years. According to this "traditional system", diseases are caused by *imbalance of prana* (a Sanskrit word for "life force" or "vital principle", the body life force). The balance of prana is determined by the three bodily quantities (doshas), viz Vata, Pitta, Kapha. The balance appears to be specific to each subject; each individual has a dominant dosha. After studying the balance of the doshas in a subject, a specific treatment-management regime is suggested and used for each patient.

Diet, herbs, massages, yoga, detoxification practices (known as "panchakarma"), oil massages, nasal lavages are all used to restore the correct balance between the body and nature. Some scientific, clinical studies have been conducted with controversial results. Some herbal combinations may include important contaminants or be poisoned by heavy metals (lead, mercury, arsenic) as they are actually considered therapeutic instruments.

Heavy-metal toxicity has been reported in a number of patients but often these practices are not officially recorded and it is difficult to find concrete data.

This "perimedical" practice or system — that requires some spiritual help — may have a questionable role when no other medicine is available or in specific contexts. It is really difficult to define its utility or efficacy in the western world and its possible connections with mainstream medicine.

Homeopathy

Homeopathy is a considered a controversial medical system, but it is an important pharmaceutical market. It is based on the principle that *like cures like.* A product, a molecule that may cause signs/symptoms of a disease at some dosages, may be effective in curing the same symptoms when administered in microscopic doses. This microscopic dose may stimulate the spontaneous healing mechanisms within the body. In theory, all homeopathy treatments are also based on the individual characteristics of the patient (considering symptoms, personality, lifestyle, health pattern).

Homeopathic remedies are obtained from some natural sources or minerals; they are given in microscopic concentrations (with the more diluted concentrations being, apparently, more effective). The dilution is so high that no molecules of the "active" product are actually found in most solutions. The bottles, basically, include water with very little evidence of any other substance. No scientific explanation has been given for this effect. No significant study has clearly shown any effect amongst several disorders.

The method moves a lot of money, has its "priests" and it has spread like a religious and philosophical belief rather than an actual proven medical technique. It is even used in some health systems — with very limited applications — without clear evidence of benefits. The producers of homeopathic remedies must specify the classification as "homeopathic", must indicate the substance included as well as its dilution. Producers must also include at least one clinical indication and instructions for safe use. It is therefore not assumed that homeopathic preparations are always biologically inactive. The FDA allows some herbal medications to be registered and labeled as homeopathic if they are prepared in specific conditions. Therefore, the original definition of homeopathic has been extended.

Actually, there is no real connection between homeopathic and herbal products. The confusion between homeopathic and herbal is often manipulated to promote questionable products. Homeopathy is used to "treat" several disorders (allergies, digestive problems, different types of pain, etc).

Controversial nonconditions and disorders (like fibromyalgia) are natural targets for homeopathy. Side effects and interactions with drugs are, of course, minimal but by using homoeopathy, some patients may delay or avoid actual medicine, sometimes with severe consequences (including death). Allergic or toxic reactions have been reported, and this remains a concern.

New Age people tend to have a strong "ideological" belief in homeopathy which often appears to be the result of resistance to or a lack of belief in the benefit gained from mainstream medicine. Some homeopathy users become "believers" in the method/system and appear to be interested more in the ideological aspects than in the technical aspects aimed at controlling medical problems. The cultural and marketing pressure behind homeopathy should not be underestimated. It is an important business and industry. It could be a criminal offence to use homeopathy in children.

Traditional Chinese medicine

According to concepts used for millennia (this is not an assurance of validity), most diseases are caused by an improper flow of the life force (*qi*). The motion of qi may be restored to its original patterns by balancing the opposite forces of *yin* and *yang* which manifest in the body as heat and cold, external and internal, deficiency and excess. Traditional Chinese procedures like acupuncture, massage, diet, medicinal herbs, meditation (*qi gong*) are used to preserve and restore qi and therefore health.

There is a vague recognition of diseases the way we see them in mainstream medicine. Chinese medicine uses traditional formulas including mixtures of herbs or herbal products to treat different disorders. Some of these traditional combinations have been studied and tested in clinical conditions. It is possible that herbal products used together may work much better than single herbal products which may be not very effective and may cause significant side effects.

At the moment, most studies are focused on single herbal products (that usually are already a mixture of several products, e.g., curcumin). Some "herbal" or natural products may be effective in treating inflammatory conditions; others are used in subjects with more serious illnesses, e.g., lung cancer (*Astrafalus*). Several Chinese herbal or natural products have been studied for hepatitis, cirrhosis and other common disorders.

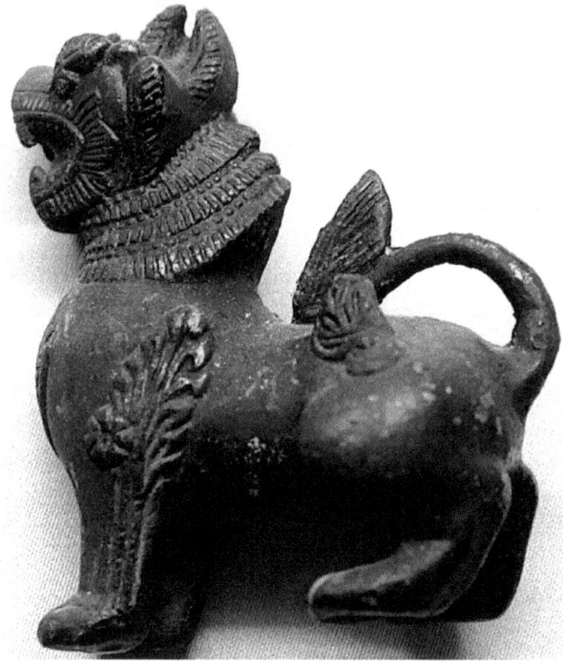

Chinese lion.

However, in this field, research is still limited. This is a result of having few sponsors. Clinical studies — if available — do not easily show the efficacy of herbal products, do not produce patents and therefore the possibility of commercially exploiting products exists.

The Chinese herbarium is very large and many products may be very active and clinically effective. These products should be recommended for proper clinical studies and (eventually) proposed in a modern pharmaceutical standard, without contaminants. With a standard dosage and with studies on absorption and metabolism, the Chinese herbarium may become a gold mine in the search for new effective products.

Without standardization, dosage and quality control, some herbal products may even kill. Also, many products may be heavily contaminated by polluted water. Some expensive products may be adulterated with cheaper, toxic substances and colorants. Some may include corticosteroids, antibiotics or other drugs and products that give them an appearance of efficacy. Pharmaceutical standards (and FDA Good Manufacturing

Practices) now enable the preparation of highly standardized products and this course of study is recommended to promote safer dosing of so-called traditional or alternative products. Clinical evaluation of some of these products in preventive or treatment studies is urgently needed.

The diagnostic processes in Chinese medicine and the physiological assumptions are difficult to fully understand, often considered questionable according to mainstream medicine, and possibly wrong or incomplete in many aspects. However, it cannot be denied that some ancient and seemingly abstract systems have produced positive health benefits for large populations for many centuries, and many products certainly must have a pharmacological basis for their actions. Traditional Chinese medicine is potentially much more useful under close supervision by expert physicians working with mainstream medicine and of course, in the right context.

Naturopathy

This method is based on the healing power of "nature". Naturopathic *practice* is based on a belief in the body's ability to heal itself through a special, invisible, intrinsic, vital energy. Naturopaths claim that the Greek physician Hippocrates from Kos was the first user of naturopathic medicine. Naturopathy has its roots in the 19th-century Natural Cure movement of Europe. Thomas Allinson started his "Hygienic Medicine" in the 1880s, promoting a natural diet in association with exercise, avoidance of the twin evils of smoking and overwork.

The name *naturopathy* was coined in 1895 by J Scheel and used by Benedict Lust, whom naturopaths consider to be the "Father of US Naturopathy". Lust had studied a form of hydrotherapy and other natural health methods in Germany with Father Sebastian Kneipp. Kneipp sent Lust to the US to *spread* his drugless method. This method includes prevention, management with a healthy lifestyle, a *whole-patient* approach and appears to rely on the natural healing abilities of the body. Finding the causes of the disease and not simply treating symptoms is also a target of this method (as it is for mainstream medicine). The method is quite comparable to other traditional healing systems (Ayurveda) and has similarities with some aspects of traditional Chinese Medicine. It is a combination of traditional therapies, medicinal herbs, homeopathy, hydrotherapy, nutrition, physical therapies (including heat and cold), now ultrasound, massage, guided imagery and stress management. At the moment, there is a strong ideology behind it.

The ideology and methods of naturopathy are based on *vitalism* and some rules of folk medicine, rather than modern, evidence-based or scientific medicine. Unfortunately, the most integral naturopathic practitioners or "healers" are against most modern medical procedures, including testing, drugs treatments, vaccinations and even surgery. Naturopathic methods rely on many unscientific notions, often leading naturopathic "doctors" to diagnoses and treatments that have no real scientific basis.

Most naturopathy *practitioners* have a strong opposition to vaccinations. The reasons for this opposition are based on the early, historical ideas which shaped the foundation of this method. A naturopathy textbook, coauthored by J Pizzorno, recalls antivaccine beliefs associated with the founding of naturopathy in the US "a return to nature in regulating the diet, breathing, exercising, bathing and the employment of various forces" *in lieu* of the smallpox vaccine. Many practitioners of naturopathic medicine have been found criminally liable in the courts of law around the world. In some countries, it is a criminal offense for naturopaths and naturopathic doctors to label themselves as medical professionals. The combination of mainstream medicine and naturopathy can be even more dangerous.

3

Mind–Body Medicine

Practitioners of mind–body medicine (MBM) uphold their belief that mental and emotional factors may influence physical health via neuronal, hormonal and immunological connections. However, this is well known in mainstream medicine. Behavioral, psychological, social and "spiritual" methods are used to preserve health and to prevent, alleviate or in some cases cure symptoms and diseases. Scientific evidence supporting a connection between body and mind is more than clear.

Management methods in mainstream medicine follow and consider the connections between physical health and the psychological implications (or causes) of medical problems and their symptoms. Techniques related to MBM include biofeedback, guided imagery, hypnotherapy, meditation and relaxation. Respiratory techniques may also be used as supportive management to alleviate chronic pain (even coronary), some aspects of ischemia, headaches, insomnia, incontinence and in facilitating childbirth. These methods are also used to help patients to cope better with problems related to chronic problems and difficult conditions (including cancer) and their consequences and also to prepare patients for surgical procedures. The evidence of some efficacy in conditions such as asthma and hypertension is very limited at the moment and needs further consideration.

Mind–body interventions include practices that use techniques designed to facilitate the mind's capacity to affect bodily function and symptoms. Imagery, meditation, hypnosis and hypnotherapy, even prayer, *art, music or dance therapy* can also be used. *The definition of therapy in this context is very wide and remains controversial.* Several mind–body interventions have shown benefits in their use within different cultural and social conditions. These methods contribute to the management or treatment in a large range of health problems.

MBM may improve the symptoms associated with chemotherapy (nausea, vomiting), improve some physical pain in patients with cancer; this improvement may be limited in time but nonetheless it may help. MBM may increase the perceived capacity to cope with significant medical problems and it may improve the overall quality of life in some patients. In addition, there is evidence supporting the influence of the brain and central nervous system upon the immune system and the capacity for some mind–body interventions to enhance immune functions, including resistance to some infection and recovery from infection and disease. This aspect is very speculative and it is very difficult to evaluate in a scientific context.

Most MBM methods are actually integrated into good mainstream medicine practices in a more complex clinical context. In conventional medicine, all mind–body interventions focus on the interaction between the brain, body and behavior and are commonly practiced in association with the main interventions (i.e., surgery or chemotherapy) with the intention of using the mind to alter or improve some physical functions and promote overall health and well-being. A strong, individual susceptibility to the use of these methods is essential for them to have any significant effect. The personality and charisma of the physician is always a significant factor in translating advice and action into useful behaviors and significant health outcomes.

Biofeedback

Biofeedback uses electronic monitoring devices to produce physiological information and parameters for the patients (heart rate, BP). Muscle tension, skin temperature, skin resistance and brain surface electrical activity are believed to be modified using biofeedback. Normal subjects and patients may use biofeedback to modify some functions or to relax, to control pain, stress, insomnia, headache, incontinence or chronic abdominal pain. Raynaud's disease (emotionally induced vasospastic conditions), attention or memory deficits (all affected by emotional factors) may also be improved. But these applications *must be* evaluated in a clinical context.

Biofeedback does not appear to be useful in asthma, but it may improve pulmonary function in some subjects. It is not clear whether through these methods (strongly affected by suggestion and personal characteristics) symptoms and conditions of *real* clinical problems are really affected by the practice or whether it is just the individual's *perception* of the problem that is affected.

Guided imagery

This method uses images to help patients relax, to promote healing and wellness (but this is not a medical condition or problem) or to improve and condition the immune system. Different forms of imagery have been used with relaxation techniques and with respiratory methods. The method may be used to manage some forms of pain and to improve the quality of life in patients with chronic diseases including cancer or patients treated with oncological therapies. Also, the consequences of psychological trauma may be improved.

Hypnotherapy

This is the most interesting of these methods; it is based on the mind–body connections. Patients (or normal subjects) are encouraged into an advanced stage of relaxation. They appear to be absorbed in the images presented by the therapist and are relatively distracted but not unconscious as they may still be influenced by the actions around them. They may be involved at different levels in their surrounding environment and in the experiences around them. Some patients may learn to autohypnotize themselves. This method — with several different variants — was previously used to treat pain, phobias and behavioral disorders; it is possible, e.g., to induce smoking cessation and weight loss in some individuals. These are not clinical conditions.

Hypnosis may control or reduce pain and anxiety, e.g., during surgery or in dental procedures. Hypnosis has been also used in the management of irritable bowel syndrome, headaches, asthma and some skin disorders where a significant component appears to be linked to stress (i.e., psoriasis). The Royal Society of Medicine in London has a specific section dealing with hypnotherapy and its clinical applications by qualified specialists. Some experiences suggest that hypnosis may be effective in lowering blood pressure. Also, it may control nausea and vomiting associated to chemotherapy. Hypnosis has also been used as a therapy in palliative cancer care. Generally, people must be susceptible to hypnosis for this method to have any measure of success. If it is to be considered a medical procedure, hypnosis requires a qualified (medical) professional and an adequate medical environment.

Meditation

Meditation may be used as an effective therapeutic aid in very limited conditions. Subjects regulate their attention and focus on some inner or external aspects of their world. Transcendental meditation and mindfulness meditation are the most studied and used methods. Meditation appears to function by producing a state of relaxation in contrast with the excessive activation of neurohormonal pathways resulting from an excess in alarm-stress response. The different methods of meditation develop a "metacognitive awareness" (described as an ability to stand back and observe the different contents and levels of consciousness).

In theory, this state of relaxation helps some subjects avoid automatic reactions to stressful situations based on definite and highly conditioned learned patterns of behavior. Meditation may help these subjects to tolerate and regulate their emotional distress. Most meditation methods have been developed within a strong religious or spiritual context and may require some isolation.

The aim of meditation was mainly associated with spiritual growth and to achieve transcendental experiences. However, some transcendental experiences were induced by so-called "masters" in highly stylized environments (isolated monasteries, high altitudes with low oxygen and with a very ascetic life) and so these apparently higher (or lower) states of consciousness may not be reproducible in a normal environment.

As a medical method, meditation, in its different forms, may give benefit to many subjects independently of spiritual or religious background, at a very limited cost and without any danger. Meditation when correctly used under supervision of qualified medical professionals may relieve anxiety, control chronic pain, manage different levels of depression or anxiety, decrease excessive stress, insomnia and also improve the perception of some chronic disorders including even cancer and cardiovascular disorders. Meditation has been sold in the perimedical market to promote "wellness" (which is not a medical concept or a physiological entity).

Method of meditation

Sit or lie in a comfortable position and determine a focus for your mind. Here are a few to consider:

- *Focus on your breath.* Breathe in and out through your nose and pay attention to some aspect of your breathing, such as the pause between breaths or the sensation of air leaving your nostrils.
- *Focus on a word, phrase or prayer.* In Transcendental Meditation, you mentally repeat a mantra, usually a Sanskrit word or sound assigned by your instructor. But you can choose your own word or mantra, such as the word *peace* (or the phrase *I want a Porsche 911*) or you can count from one to four over and over again. You can also coordinate your mantra with your breathing.
- *Focus on the moment.* This is also known as mindfulness meditation. You become aware of sensations, sounds and thoughts. You simply notice them and let them go. Or you may notice the sensations in your body — stomach growling or thigh cramping. Or, you may think you do.
- Many people meditate with their eyes closed. Others prefer to keep their eyes partially open with a soft focus. It doesn't matter whether you lie down or sit on the floor, a chair, a meditation cushion or a bench, as long as you're comfortable. But don't get too comfortable; you may fall asleep.
- Start with 5-min meditation sessions once or twice a day and work up to 20-min sessions.

Relaxation techniques

Relaxation techniques are used to relieve tension by reducing the activity of the sympathetic nervous system. Susceptibility and individual perception are very important to obtain results by these methods. Relaxation methods have been used to lower blood pressure (the effects may be only limited in time). Relaxation techniques are also used to decrease muscle tension and to slow down metabolic processes. Relaxation may be also visible in brain wave activity. All relaxation techniques are generally used in association with other "physiological" methods including meditation, guided imagery, hypnotherapy, respiratory exercise. All methods are generally safe and have very limited costs, but there are only a few studies showing their activity and efficacy. The individual capacity, patience and attention required to use these techniques is an important component, but this is instrumental in limiting their usefulness. The people able to meditate and relax are possibly the individuals that do not need these methods.

Yoga

Yoga is an ancient practice — it is not a medical tool — that aims to induce physical, mental and spiritual *well-being* through a combination of postures (asanas), breathing techniques and meditation. This practice is increasingly popular among people seeking relaxation, a spiritual path or improvements in flexibility, coordination, balance, strength and endurance. It is also cool at the moment.

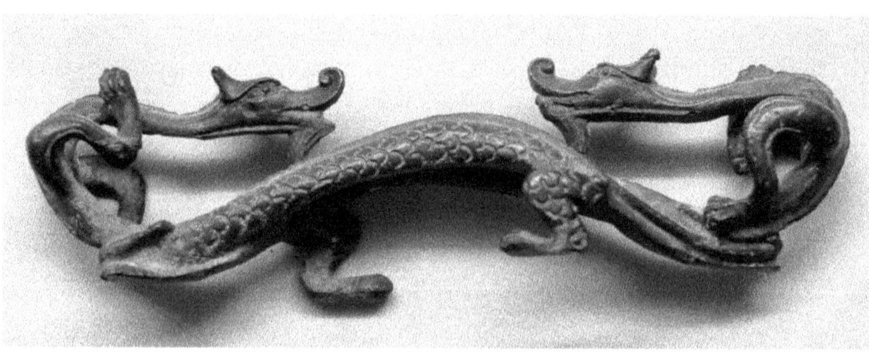

Two dragons.

Yoga may ease arthritis, help people stop smoking and improve some of the symptoms of carpal tunnel syndrome (but this seems too optimistic). Other benefits of yoga, when practiced regularly, may include reduced anxiety, slowed breathing, lowered blood pressure, altered brainwaves and (there is no evidence) more efficient heart blood flow (for what it means). It is claimed that yoga can treat specific mental and physical disorders, but real controlled studies are not yet in sufficient quantities to support such claims.

At the very least, yoga can be relaxing and may improve physical conditioning. An experienced instructor who adapts postures to levels of flexibility is likely to help rather than harm. But yoga requires some discipline and concentration. It is not an "easy fix". There are different types of yoga, but no medical meaning has been assigned to any of them due to a lack of clinically reproducible evidence.

Tai chi

Designed to foster the free flow of energy (chi) that *practitioners* believe is necessary for good health, tai chi was developed as a martial art in China more than 1,000 years ago. Tai chi is based on a series of slow, flowing movements that resemble a dance. Tai chi is used today to gain emotional and physical balance, reduce stress and strengthen muscles and joints. Because it can help with alertness and tranquility, some people use it as a form of movement-controlled meditation. Also it is a good choice if you want to avoid real exercise.

Tai chi comprises hundreds of combinations of continuous movements that require concentration, balance and grace (and some patience). When combined with deep, rhythmic breathing, these movements can increase your circulation (this is just an assumption that does not have a medical meaning), relax your mind and body and, possibly, ease chronic pain. Practicing tai chi has also been shown to improve balance, reduce falls and reduce the risk of fractures.

4

Biologically Based Practices

Natural occurring substances (e.g., shark cartilage, glucosamine, etc.), diet-based therapy, the use of herbal products (not in pharmaceutical standards), "orthomolecular" medicine and chelation therapy are all considered as biologically based practices (BBPs).

Diets and dietary therapy

It is important to consider that no diet is a therapy or a substitute for a therapy or constitutes a real therapeutic measure. Any diet may have a preventive value, may help patients to improve; it may have a broad therapeutic value, but generally, it cannot be used as a single therapy.

Macrobiotic diet

Macrobiotic diet has been considered a fad, trendy diet (albeit now a bit "out of fashion") fixed on some ideas about types of food derived from Zen Buddhism. The original macrobiotic diet pretends to balance the yin and yang elements of food and requires specific "healthy" cookware. The principles of macrobiotic diets are planned around a reduction of animal products, eating locally grown foods that are used according to seasonal availability; this diet also requires the eating of meals in moderation.

Macrobiotics experts claim that this diet is helpful for people with cancer and other chronic diseases, but there is no evidence to support these suggestions. The diet if extreme may even be nutritionally harmful and kill.

Studies indicating results of the use of this diet for long periods are limited and fragmented. The American Cancer Society and Cancer Research UK *do not* recommend this diet for cancer patients. Suggestions that a macrobiotic diet improves cardiovascular disease and diabetes appear quite logical but are not easily demonstrable. The diet corresponds partially to the most common scientific, dietary approaches suggested in the prevention of cardiovascular disease; that is, it is low in fats and calories, involves eating in moderation, is boring, etc.

Most macrobiotic diets are not nutritionally complete and some subjects following a strict macrobiotic diet are at increased risk of developing scurvy. One of the earlier, extreme macrobiotic diets (in which it was suggested to eat only brown rice and drink only water) has been linked to severe nutritional deficiencies and even deaths. Strict macrobiotic diets that include no animal products may result in important nutritional deficiencies unless they are carefully planned and individually studied. The danger may be more important for patients with oncological conditions who may be affected by severe, unwanted weight loss and sarcopenia. These patients often have *increased* nutritional and caloric requirements. The use of only a macrobiotic diet as a type of treatment for cancer and for the avoidance or delay of conventional medical care for oncological conditions is likely to have serious health consequences. Such nutritional imbalances are likely to be more exacerbated in children and pregnant or breastfeeding women.

The specific rules of this type of diet (approaching a form of ritual) may state that cooking utensils should be made only from defined, "healthy" materials such as wood or glass. Avoidance of potentially "contaminating" materials, including plastic, copper and pans with nonstick coatings, is encouraged.

Brown rice and other whole grains such as barley, millet, oats, quinoa, spelt, rye, and teff (Williams lovegrass or annual bunch grass) are considered by macrobiotic followers to be the foods in which *yin* and *yang* are likely to be effectively balanced. Therefore, lists of macrobiotic foods that define a food as yin or yang generally compare them to whole grains. Nightshade vegetables, which include tomatoes, peppers, potatoes and eggplant, are considered extremely yin. Spinach, beets and avocados are not recommended or are used with limitations in most macrobiotic cooking. Some macrobiotic "practitioners" also discourage the use of nightshades because they include the alkaloid solanine, thought to affect calcium balance. Some adherents to macrobiotic diets believe that nightshade vegetables can cause inflammation in the body and even osteoporosis, but there is no evidence of this as yet.

Gerson therapy or Gerson method

Gerson therapy or Gerson method is a particularly dangerous form of cancer management invented by Dr. Gerson. The "therapy" claims that cancer is caused by "toxins" in food that creates an imbalance of potassium and sodium in the body. The alleged method for "curing" this problem is an extremely *low sodium + high potassium* diet including lots of juice, raw, organic fruits and vegetables, massive amounts of vitamin supplements and enemas of coffee, castor oil, hydrogen peroxide or ozone. This treatment is supposed to flush out "toxins" and "repair" internal organs, particularly the liver.

Most of the "research" supporting the therapy is anecdotal, including some cases studied by the author. The National Cancer Institute reviewed some of his case studies and found the method to be ineffective. The American Cancer Society has issued warnings that the method can be harmful. There have been reports of comas, seizures, and death resulting from extremely low sodium levels and imbalance of electrolytes in the patients undergoing the "therapy". The diet has been blamed for the death and faster death of patients who substituted it for standard medical care.

The Pritikin diet

The Pritikin diet is a low-fat, high-fiber diet which forms part of the "Pritikin Program for Diet and Exercise", a lifestyle regimen originally created by N. Pritikin. The diet is based on a low-fat, high-fiber food and on the limitation of red meat, alcohol and processed food. When it was launched, the diet was considered radical, but its precepts are now considered largely in alignment with common, mainstream, nutritional advices.

The Pritikin diet has been categorized as a fad diet with serious and important disadvantages including a very boring food choice, flatulence and the risk of feeling almost always too hungry. A fad diet or *diet cult* is a diet that makes promises of weight loss or other health advantages such as *longer life* without solid scientific backing. In many cases, these diets are characterized by highly restrictive or unusual food choices. Celebrity endorsements are frequently used to promote fad diets, which may generate significant revenue for the creators, particularly from the sale of associated products. These diets have been used with the claim of treating or preventing diseases (cancer, cardiovascular disorders) or to generally promote wellness (always remembering that "wellness" is not a clinical condition, is not a physiological condition and basically is nothing).

For a warrior, "wellness" may be in a battle. For a poet, it may be a peaceful spot to write poems. For a physician, it may be a chaotic moment, in a busy emergency unit, with screaming people, saving lives.

The Mediterranean diet

The Mediterranean diet is now commonly accepted (possibly too overrated) as most of the benefits are due to lifestyle, not only food.

The Ornish diet

The Ornish diet (very low-fat vegetarian diet) theoretically can help reverse arterial plaques that cause coronary artery disease, slow down the progression of atherosclerosis or prostate and other cancers. This diet would probably be an improvement on the most common current Western or American diet if people could actually follow it for long periods of time, for decades. But its claims about the dangers of saturated fat and red meat probably go well beyond science and in some cases contradict it. Often, it is not the product but the quantity which constitutes a significant risk element.

Macrobiotic diets have anecdotally reported cancer remission, but this has also been reported by patients attending Lourdes. Diets require long periods of observations and a cultural and environmental background (including the growth and use of the things being used as food and a parallel lifestyle). Diets cannot be used as a miracle therapy alone.

Orthomolecular medicine

Orthomolecular medicine is a form of alternative medicine, aiming to maintain human health through artificial nutritional supplementation. The concept of the diet is elaborated around the idea of an optimum nutritional environment in the body and suggests that diseases may reflect theoretical deficiencies in this environment. Treatments for diseases, according to this view, involve attempts to correct imbalances or deficiencies based on individual biochemistry, by the daily use of active substances such as vitamins, minerals, amino acids, trace elements and fatty acids.

The notions behind orthomolecular medicine are not presently supported by any medical evidence; as a therapy, the diet is not effective. Even the accuracy of calling the orthomolecular approach a form of medicine has been questioned. The misleading information that something is a therapy is very confusing for many individuals. Diets and nutritional methods are not therapies and, so far, cannot even be considered preventive methods as there are only limited results. The approach of orthomolecular medicine consists of a megavitamin therapy. Its practice evolved through the use of dosage of vitamins and minerals many times higher than the recommended dietary intake. Orthomolecular fans may also incorporate a variety of other styles of nutritional management into their approaches, including some dietary restrictions, megadoses of nonvitamin nutrients and even mainstream pharmaceutical drugs often used out of their prescription limits.

Diet gurus argue that nonoptimal levels of certain substances can cause health issues beyond simple vitamin deficiency and see the balance of these substances as an integral part of health management. Linus Pauling invented the term and concept of “orthomolecular” (the right molecules in the right amounts). Gurus of orthomolecular medicine indicate that treatment plans must be based on each patient's individual biochemistry. This nutritional "medical" approach provides what are considered optimal doses of substances that are present naturally in the body. In theory, the use of supradietary doses of micronutrients, high doses of vitamins, minerals, enzymes, hormones (melatonin), amino acids, combination of elements and products used to modulate inflammation and degenerative processes may produce benefits in cancer, cardiovascular diseases, chronic fatigue syndrome and chronic pain, even autism or psychiatric conditions. However, studies are very limited and very controversial. It has been suggested that high doses of micronutrients may cause side effects or increase some incidence of cancers. If you have normal levels, it is very difficult to make you more normal and give you any real benefit.

Other nutritional elements

Fish oil (FO) derivatives have an important logic and have been used to control hypertrigliceridemia, inflammatory conditions and even mood disorders (this is an aspect very difficult to show). High doses of antioxidants have been used to prevent macular degeneration and a high dose of melatonin has been used in attempts to prevent or treat cancer (no evidence available). When and if evidence is collected in a specific condition, most of these management methods generally become an integral part of mainstream medicine. FO products are used to control platelet aggregation and lipids in patients that cannot use antiplatelet agents or statins. There are very good studies and more are in progress.

Chelation therapy

The standardized use of chelation in mainstream, standard medicine is specifically reserved to metal poisoning. In this approach, a drug is used to bind and remove from the body an excess of toxic metals or minerals (lead, calcium, copper, iron). Chelation with EDTA is used to remove calcium and to treat atherosclerosis; there is really no evidence about the clinical efficacy or safety of this method.

Calcified plaques in atherosclerotic arteries are basically nonmetabolically active. These plaques are dead tissue with almost no circulation. It is very difficult to produce changes in them. Also, calcification in atherosclerotic plaques is a late observation. The dangerous removal of calcium may even produce a loss of stability of the plaque making them more prone to rupture, thrombosis and embolization.

5

Manipulative Body-Based Practice

Methods in this practice may include the following:

- Chiropractic,
- Massage therapy,
- Reflexology,
- Structural integration.

Chiropractic

This well-defined method (with undefined perimedical borders) seeks to treat and correct the relationship between the structure and position of the spine and the functions of the nervous system. This element is considered the key to restore "health". The main method in this technique is spinal manipulation. But chiropractors also use different (costly) types of physical therapy (heat, cold, electrical stimulation, rehabilitation strategies, massage, acupressure) with exercise and lifestyle changes.

The effects are generally a short-term relief of symptoms, particularly of lower back pain. The real efficacy for back pain is still very unclear. The method has been used in patients with headache (but data are considered not reliable), neck pain and other forms of pain (e.g., due to nerve compression). The efficacy of several different applications — including nonmusculoskeletal problems — is still unclear.

Rare, adverse effects and complications may be caused by chiropractic therapy, particularly from manual manipulation which may damage arteries or veins (e.g., at the neck). In patients with osteoporosis or neuropathy, chiropractic is not recommended and it is considered unsafe in subjects with strokes, after spinal surgery or in patients with vascular disorders and coagulation problems. *Individual ability of the chiropractor is a determinant factor in determining the success of the treatment.*

Massage as a therapy

Massage with different methods may reduce pain, stress and tension. Massage may have a therapeutic value for muscoloskeletal symptoms and for stress (this is not a clinical condition), and it is widely accepted. It may also help to relieve muscle soreness, pain due to back injuries, fibromyalgia, anxiety, fatigue, pain, nausea and vomiting in cancer patients. Low-birth-weight infants have been treated with massage to improve their reactivity and growth. Massage may also relieve constipation and control asthma (but studies are very limited).

Side effects — excluding costs — may include bruising and bleeding in subjects with low platelet count, subjects using anticoagulants or subjects with coagulation problems. Pressure should not be applied on bones with osteoporosis or metastases, and massage of thrombotic legs should never be attempted by any other than qualified medical personnel. All these applications should always be under close medical supervision. Medical advice and approval is always essential before management.

Massage is very diffuse and widely accepted; it may have an efficacy in most patients and is closely linked to the abilities of the operators. Massage has also many formats. For instance, *Shiatsu* is a form of Japanese bodywork based on ideas developed in the framework of the traditional Chinese medicine. There is no evidence that *shiatsu* is an effective medical treatment. Still, many subjects claim to have benefits and the method is widely used in different contexts, often in subjects with minimal medical problems.

Reflexology

In this method, manual therapy is applied to specific areas of the foot. These areas correspond to different parts of the body via *meridians*. The stimulation which is quite comparable to acupuncture may eliminate "blocks of energy", considered to be responsible for pain or disease in the corresponding body parts. The method has been used in different applications, e.g., to relieve anxiety in patients with cancer, and in other applications.

At the moment, there is no convincing evidence that reflexology is effective for any medical condition. Users of this method claim that the feet and hands are especially sensitive and that reflexologists have mapped the entire body into "reflexes" on the feet, renaming "zone therapy" as reflexology. Reflexologists mostly use techniques developed by the reflexologist Laura Norman. Clinical applications are uncertain, but some people benefit from the method on an individual basis.

Structural integration

This is a technique including deep massage intended to help in the realignment of the body by altering the length and tone of myofascial (muscle) tissues. The basis of this technique is the belief that misalignment of myofascial tissues, resulting from improper posture and emotional and physical traumas, may have a detrimental effect on a person's "energy" level, self-image, muscular efficiency, perceptions and general health.

This method is also called Rolfing. It is based on Ida Rolf's ideas about how the human body's "energy field" can benefit when aligned with the Earth's gravitational field. So it would probably not work in space or on Mars. Biologist Dan Agin has identified Rolfing as a popular kind of "quack medicine" in the "raucous bazaar" of the US's alternative medicine scene (which is quite crowded at the moment).

Good health is believed to be due to correct body alignment. This form of deep tissue manipulation tends to correct alignment and depends on specific manipulations of muscles and their fasciae. The technique is clinically unproven and often quite painful.

Other therapies

Cupping, scraping, and moxibustion are seen as very *controversial* methods. They may cause lesions that may be mistaken for abuse, particularly in children. *These methods are supposed to* stimulate the body's energy — quite in line with acupuncture — enabling presumed "toxins" to leave the body.

In *cupping*, air is heated in a cup that is placed onto the skin. The suction from the cup, which is kept in place for minutes, has been used to treat pain, bronchitis, asthma and intestinal disorders. Lesions to the skin (from the heated cups) are possible. The method has no documented evidence of clinical activity so far.

Scraping is used to treat cold, flu, muscular pain, stiffness. A coin or a spoon may be used to rub the skin on the back, neck and shoulders. It's incredible to believe, but I have heard of "healers" using (I guess expired) credit cards. Some linear scars and ecchymosis are possible. Its clinical efficacy is unknown so far and seems very difficult to show in studies.

In *moxibustion* (named from the herb moxa), a mixture of herbs is burned close to the skin or onto the skin over some acupuncture points. Herbs are also used as incense sticks. Fever, pain, arthritis, digestive problems may be "treated" and improved. Some applications may cause burns and papular or bullous lesions.

6

Energy Medicine

According to "experts", this "nonmedicine" relies upon the manipulation of energy fields (or biofields). The presumed therapy is based on the belief that universal life forces of subtle energy reside in and around the body. Qi gong, used in traditional Chinese medicine, is considered an energy therapy.

Acupuncture

Acupuncture (AP) is a very diffuse therapy which is included within the Chinese traditional medicine. Specific points on the body are stimulated by needles placed into the skin and in the underlying tissues. According to traditional explanations, the stimulations unblock the flow of qi along some energy pathways (meridians) and are believed to restore balance. More physiological explanations may be possible. More than 350 AP points are located along the meridians. The procedures are not painful but may cause some tingling sensations. The stimulations and their effects may be increased by twisting or warming the needles. Appropriate points can be stimulated by pressure (acupressure), lasers, ultrasound, low-voltage current (electroacupuncture) applied to the needle.

AP releases various neurotransmitters (endorphins) which act as painkillers. The efficacy — limited — has been documented for applications in which AP is used as a pain reliever, an antinausea or antiemetic. Results of studies comparing sham AP and real AP seem to produce comparable results. However, AP may relieve some vasomotor symptoms, may improve lung function in patients with asthma and may relieve pain. AP has been used as a significant aid in anesthesiology. In weight loss or smoking cessation (these are not medical conditions), AP seems to have no effects or minimal activity. The evidence so far is mixed.

Acupuncture steps

Following are the steps in AP procedure:

- From 1 to 20 or more hair-thick needles are inserted under the skin.
- Some may go in as deep as 3–6 cm, depending on where they're placed and what the treatment is for. Other needles are placed superficially.
- The needles usually are left in the tissues for 15–30 min.
- Little or no pain results from insertion. Significant pain is a sign that the procedure has been done improperly.
- Once inserted, the needles may be moved gently by hand or stimulated with an electrical current or heat.
- Several sessions are needed. Relief from the first one is uncommon but if nothing's happening after six or eight sessions, then AP probably isn't for you. You have to pay anyway.
- If there is some relief, you may consider it as a chance.
- It could take months to alleviate pain, and pain, in months, may disappear spontaneously.

Side effects of AP (including infections) are generally limited when the method is correctly used by real experts. Worsening of symptoms and vasovagal symptoms are the most common complaints after AP. Fainting or drowsiness is possible and patients should be supine, at least for the initial treatment. Viral infections — described in the past — are rare as disposable needles are now used.

- AP should not be used in patients with bleeding disorders.
- Electroacupuncture should not be used in subjects with pacemakers or implanted defibrillators.

AP may stimulate uterine contractions, and in traditional Chinese medicine, it has been used to regulate labor. Specially trained practitioners should use AP in pregnant women only in cases where it is needed. Lengthy training and practice is required to get appropriate methodology and results with some clinical or periclinical value.

AP should only be used by physicians or by experts under close medical supervision. The method, globally, deserves more attention, research and further studies. In most subjects, it appears to produce minor relief of minor problems and symptoms at low cost and without side effects.

Magnets

Magnets are popular treatments for musculoskeletal disorders. Magnotherapy is considered a pseudoscientific alternative medicine method, generally involving the use of static magnetic fields. Most studies of magnotherapy have shown no efficacy on pain relief or on body structures and organs. Static, permanent magnets may relieve some pain in osteoarthritis, but there is limited evidence to back this up. Pulsating electromagnetic fields may produce faster healing of nonunion fractures, but standards for these applications are still uncertain. The most common supposed mechanism of the action of magnets is an improvement in blood flow in the tissues in the magnetic field. However, the magnetic field produced by most therapeutic devices is too weak to affect hemoglobin and other blood and tissue components (muscle, bones, blood vessels or organs).

Contraindications for the use of magnetic treatments are pregnancy, the presence of implanted cardiac devices (pacemakers), insulin pumps and the use of patches releasing drugs. The physical and biological claims of magnetic therapies are still unproven, and so far, no definite effects on health or healing have been established. Although hemoglobin is weakly diamagnetic (when oxygenated) or paramagnetic (when deoxygenated), the magnets used in magnetic therapy are too weak to have any significant measurable effect (either physiological or clinical) on the microcirculation.

The worldwide magnotherapy industry moves a market of over a billion dollars per year (some 300 million per year in the US alone). A US National Science Foundation report on public attitudes and understanding of science noted that magnotherapy is "not at all scientific". Most producers of equipment and therapists make claims about magnotherapy by using pseudoscientific and fashionable new-age language. However, their claims are not supported by studies.

Therapeutic touch

In this method, therapists use their "healing energy" to identify and repair "imbalance" in patients' *biofields.* Therapists do not touch their patients but move their hands over the patients using their healing powers. The method has been used to lessen anxiety and to improve a sense of well-being in some patients with cancer. The effects have not been studied in depth and appear really difficult to evaluate or even to have a logical background.

There is no good medical evidence for the effectiveness of therapeutic touch (although it has to be said that there is no *bad* evidence either). A Cochrane systematic review found that there was no significant evidence that therapeutic touch promotes healing of acute wounds. It is actually surprising to see that the Cochrane "dark" shadow involves even these esoteric healing practices. The American Cancer Society has also indicated that there is no scientific evidence supporting any claims that therapeutic touch can cure cancer or other diseases.

Reiki

This is a comparable "fluid" method which allegedly originated in Japan. The therapist channels some energy through their hands and transfers this energy into the patient's body, thereby promoting some form of healing. The therapist in this case appears to have some special healing powers that are required for these treatments. Reiki has been adapted into varying cultural traditions. *Palm healing* or *hands-on healing* via some "universal energy" is allegedly transferred to encourage emotional or physical healing.

Reiki is considered pseudoscience. It is based on *qi*, which practitioners define is a universal life force, although there is no remote evidence that such a life force exists. Clinical research has not shown any effect of Reiki: it is not a medical treatment usable for any medical condition. However, some patients claim individual benefits.

7
Conclusion

In consideration of the whole universe of CAM, some institutions have developed centers for alternative or complementary medicine to satisfy their patients or customers who are willing to try them. These centers, predominantly staffed with qualified medical personnel, ensure that even these methods are used under safe conditions and when required, in association with more tested conventional methods of mainstream medicine and treatment.

Most treatment methods border witchcraft. Definitions of witchcraft are as follows:

- the use of sorcery or magic,
- communication with the devil or with a familiar,
- an irresistible influence or fascination.

Luckily for healers, the number of idiots or selective idiots born on the planet is still relatively high, so they will have some business for a long period of time. Some of the "practices" are wildly superior to the inventions of G. Lucas, and many subjects are really unable to separate a gray reality from an apparently shining unreality.

The system of the barefoot doctors

The Chinese experiment

Complementary, alternative and supportive–supplementary medicine integrated with modern medicine in a socialized system

This is by far the most interesting and comprehensive system developed to blend alternative–complementary methods. It is mainly based on traditional Chinese medicine, supplementary medicine and modern medical methods.

Barefoot doctors (BDs) (Chinese: 赤脚医生; pinyin: *chìjiǎo yīshēng*) were farmers who received minimal and very basic medical and/or paramedical training and worked in rural areas and villages in China where no physician was available. Their purpose was to take concepts of healthcare and social medicine to rural areas where urban-trained doctors, accustomed to having a hospital as a reference point of care-giving, would not settle. BDs promoted simple, basic hygiene, preventive healthcare and family planning and treated the common illnesses and medical problems. The name comes from southern farmers, who would often work barefoot in the rice paddies.

In the 1930s, the Rural Reconstruction Movement had pioneered the presence of village health workers trained in basic health as part of a coordinated system. There had been provincial experiments after 1949, but after Mao Zedong's healthcare speech in 1965 the concept was developed and institutionalized. In his speech, Mao Zedong criticized the urban bias of the Chinese medical system of the time and had called for a system with greater focus on the well-being of the rural population at the most basic level. Actually, most of these concepts were also used to support Obamacare. Most of these Chinese villagers and rural population lived in remote locations, far away from hospitals and cities; China's health policy changed quickly after this speech.

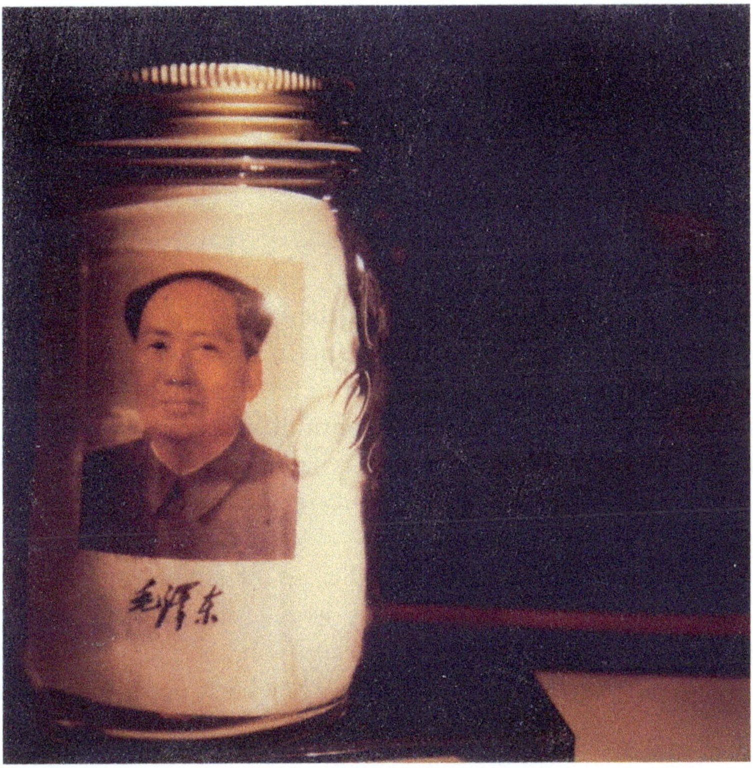

Mao's historical role ends. His indications can be put in a jar and stored.

After 1968, the BDs program became integrated into the national health policy also assuming an iconic political value and showing the interest of the politicians for the more excluded part of the population. "Rural" and "poor" at the time were almost synonyms. These programs were called "rural cooperative medical systems" (RCMS) and had the aim of including the participation of the community with the rural provision of health services. BDs became a part of the Cultural Revolution, which also radically diminished the influence of the Ministry of Health, which was dominated — at the time — by West-trained doctors.

Regarding training, BDs usually graduated from secondary school and then received about 6 months of training, including some basic surgical skill also, at a county or community hospital. Training length varied from a few months to 1½ y. Training was focused on the most common local problems including epidemic disease prevention, managing or curing simple problems or diseases that were frequent observations in the specific area. BDs were trained to use modern Western medicines (antibiotics, antiseptics) and techniques.

An important (distorted) part of the Cultural Revolution was the movement of sending "intellectuals", and in this case, doctors, to serve in the countryside or in poor, rural or remote areas. They would live in an area for half a year to a year and continue and improve the education of the BDs. About a fifth of the BDs later entered a formal medical school. BDs acted as primary healthcare providers at the most basic levels.

BDs — as a system — included a set of simple medicines, both Western and Chinese, that the BDs would dispense after diagnosis. Often, they grew their own medicinal herbs and prepared some complementary treatments in their backyard. They basically tried to integrate

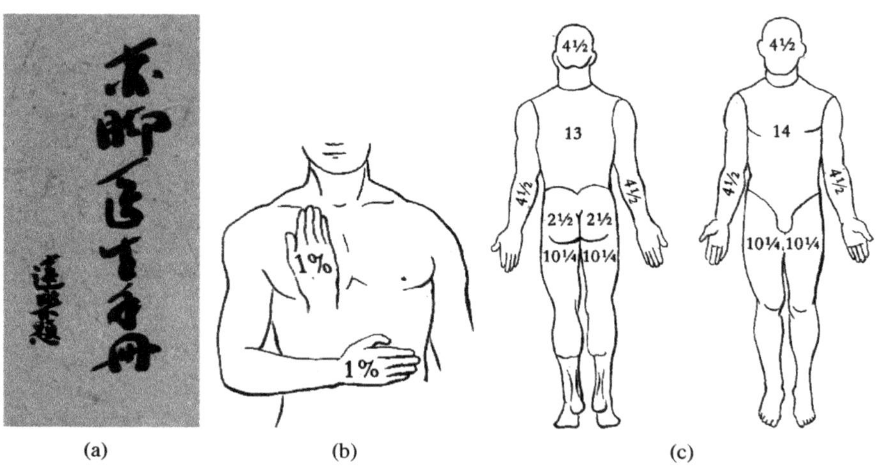

(a) (b) (c)

(a) BDs, (b) the Palmar method and (c) new nine-division method.

principles and methods of both modern Western and traditional Chinese medicine including acupuncture (very well accepted by the rural populations).

BDs were also actively involved in rural and farm work, often spending about half of their time on these activities. The rural farmers perceived them as their peers and respected their advice more as they saw the BDs as a part of their life and community. The BDs were integrated into a system where they could refer seriously ill people or patients not treatable by their limited "clinics" to main, modern hospitals. BDs provided mostly primary healthcare services focused mainly on prevention and education more than treatments. Also, BDs provided most basic immunizations, helped in "normal" delivery for pregnant women and improved the basic sanitation and hygiene in villages and schools.

The income of the BDs was calculated as if it were agricultural work; they were paid roughly half of what a classically trained doctor made in China at the time. The funding to pay BDs came from the community, from collective welfare funds as well as from local farmer contributions. This program was successful in part because the doctors were selected and paid by their own villages. By the 1960s, there were RCMS programs in some 90% of China's rural villages.

According to several reports, the work of the BDs in some 10 y effectively reduced healthcare costs in China and provided primary care and treatments to a rural farming population that had very limited access to medical services. The program was — apparently — very cost effective. The World Health Organization (WHO) regarded RCMS as a "successful example of solving shortages or medical services in rural areas". The system of the BDs, providing primary, often very primary, healthcare was considered effective and the basic healthcare became an affordable cost for a very large number of people. This system, considered very innovative and quite revolutionary at the time, gave China the right for admission into the United Nations (UN) and WHO. It was considered an example of a system capable of controlling disease in poor countries with simple, systematic, adequate often low-technological solutions, and also blending some selected traditional, local, simple medical solutions with modern medical concepts.

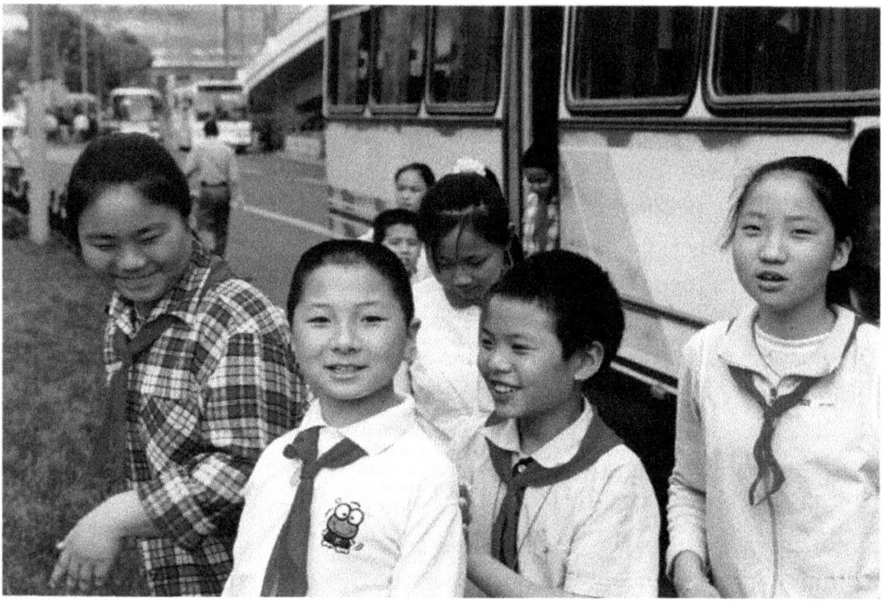

Within the groove of the Cultural Revolution, the global effort of barefoot medicine was also aimed to fight all the "useless" traditional negative practices and superstitions — part of many local ways of managing diseases, bordering witchcraft — that were plaguing the rural culture of the time. Superstitions were separated from medical practices, and again in the full process of the Cultural Revolution, the word "traditional" acquired a sinister and dark meaning.

The end of the age of the BDs in China coincided with an improvement in quality of life and in a progressive evolution from the hard, isolated, rural poverty of some villages to an industrial evolution and urbanization with improvement in communications. Also, nutritional factors, economy and education had been greatly improved, and there was no need anymore for very low-level solutions to very small problems basically linked to poverty and very hard life.

Some two-thirds of the village doctors currently practicing in the present rural China began their training as a BD. This includes, for instance, Dr. Chen Zhu who became the Minister of Health after practicing as a BD for 5 y (before completing additional medical training). The BD system was abolished in 1981 with the end of the commune system of agricultural cooperatives. The changes in Chinese economy with improvements in conditions and communications caused a change towards a partial privatization of the medical system which could not sustain the BDs as a diffuse system.

The BDs had a chance to take a national exam to formally become village doctors. Those BDs that did not pass the exam — unless old — would be employed as village health aides. Village doctors began charging most patients for most of their services (very low fees), and with the new economic situation, they began to shift their attention more to treatments for chronic conditions and drugs rather than preventive methods, education and generally improving community health.

By 1984, village RCMS coverage had decreased from 90% of the villages to less than 5%. In 1989, the Chinese government tried to partially restore a cooperative healthcare system in the most rural areas by launching a capillary, national primary healthcare program. This effort increased the coverage of the system to some 10% of the population (that is a big number in China, around some 140 millions) by 1993. In 1994, the government established what is defined as "The Program", an effort to re-establish a system of primary healthcare coverage for the rural population.

In 2003, the Chinese government proposed a new "cooperative" medical system operated and funded by the government. This program is run more like an insurance program (the cost is approximately 10 Renminbi/year for each person covered by the program) and even covers people with serious diseases and conditions. This new program relies heavily upon the lessons learned from the times of the BDs — which were completely different with a more diffuse and radical poverty — but it still faces many challenges in providing sufficient, cost-effective care for China's rural populations. The system associating some revised "traditional Chinese Medicine" and modern, standard medicine make the whole system a very interesting and a possible model for complementary/alternative and supplementary medical methods.

It must be considered that only China has these sort of numbers: a population of some 1.403 500 365 in 9,596,961 km^2 (with about 90% of Han and more than 55 ethnic groups). The system of the BDs was among the most important inspirations for the WHO conference in Alma-Ata,

Kazakhstan, in 1978. The Alma-Ata Declaration was signed unanimously and considered a revolutionary breakthrough in international health philosophy and planning. The document called for the involvement of the local communities in deciding healthcare priorities, called for an emphasis on primary and preventive healthcare and most importantly tried to link medicine with trade, economics, industry, rural politics and other political and social areas.

International development with NGOs

In 1977, Jean-Pierre Willem created an international humanitarian apolitical nongovernmental organization (NGO) of doctors called *Médecins aux pieds nus* in France. Volunteers worked in Burundi, Colombia and Southeast Asia with some local healers to develop "medical gardens" for plants of medical value and to produce usable and standard supplements from these plants. This NGO leads ethnobiological missions based on "proximity, prevention and humility".

The influence of the BDs philosophy can be found in many medical systems and healthcare systems in many countries. It was clear that many problems should be addressed and solved with prevention and community work. Many researchers left hospital to work in wider communities to study prevention, particularly cardiovascular prevention. For instance, the connection between the Framingham study and the diffuse preventive methods of the BD seems vague and nondirect, but there are significant similarities in totally different social and medical contexts.

Our epidemiological studies in Central Italy (San Valentino, Umbria and other places) and equivalent studies in UK, Finland and Cyprus were pushed by the need to study patients before they were patients in their actual environment. Many doctors — mainly used to working in big university hospitals — left the health castles and started to work applying local screening and prevention in small villages. The concept that "we are good doctors if many patients do not need to go to the hospitals" became a significant part of modern cardiovascular medicine, well recognized by the American Heart Association which established definite sections (i.e., population studies) to deal with preventive cardiovascular activities.

The lesson of the BDs is still in need of a full scientific and technical evaluation, without recourse to the surrounding ideology but focusing on the cost and efficacy of small, fast and cheap interventions, particularly those with a preventive value and a local geography, close to the patients or to groups of would-be patients. The ideology of politicians blended with the pragmatism of the real doctors created in the largest medical experimental effort in history is still not fully recognized for political assumptions. It is difficult to believe, but some concepts derived by this form of diffuse, socialized medicine can be also found in the Obamacare documents.[a]

[a] See *A Barefoot Doctor's Manual: A Concise Edition of the Classic Work of Eastern Herbal Medicine* by Hunan Zhong, Yi Yao Yan, Jau Suo, Ge Wei Hui (Running Press, 2002) and *Il Cuore Della Medicina* by G. Belcaro (Un libro rivoluzion.ario).

Part 2
Pharma-Standard Supplements

1

Introduction

Introduction by Prof. G. Appendino

Plant-based medicine has never been static and oriented to the past. On the contrary, it has always benefited from technological advances. Thus, the discovery of distillation replaced fumigations with essential oils and complemented water-based preparations like teas and decoctions with alcohol preparations like elixirs.

The spectacular advances in the realm of phytochemistry and molecular biology have substantially replaced medicinal plants and the simple kitchen-style preparations thereof (decoctions, teas) with standardized extracts and drug-inspired formulations. Ideally, an extract should preserve and magnify the activity of a plant in terms of potency, at the same time minimizing its side effects (miracle cures devoid of side effects are an abstraction). To this purpose, standardization, i.e., knowledge on the nature and the concentration of specific compounds, is of critical relevance.

Botanical extracts act because they contain specific compounds that modulate certain metabolic or physiological networks in a specific way, generally acting on several end points and in combination. Reducing the activity of botanical extracts to a single constituent is derogatory for plant-based medicine. If activity can indeed be related to a specific constituent, it will be more reasonable to use it as a pure compound as has been done for the so-called heroic drugs, i.e., a plant whose activity for a specific condition is essentially due to a specific constituent. Opium has nowadays been replaced by morphine, belladonna by atropine, and foxglove by its purified saponins.

On the other hand, the activity of most medicinal plants cannot be traced back to a single constituent and mechanism of action and instead results from the combined action of a bouquet of constituents and a bouquet of mechanisms. Just like vanilla smells much better than vanillin, extracts are often better than their single constituents in terms of potency, tolerability or both. Hemp-based medicine is a striking example. Pure tetrahydrocannabinol (THC) as an antiemetic agent has a low compliance in patients because of its psychotropic and anxiogenic activity. Patients prefer marijuana because another cannabinoid, cannabidiol (CBD), moderates the side effects of THC and complements its activity.

In plant medicine, the mathematic relationships are skewed, and 2 + 2 does not generally mean 4. So, gingko is not ginkgolides or flavonoids but a combination of the two; curcumin is not molecular curcumin but a combination of three curcuminoids; *Boswellia* is not a single triterpenoid acid like acetyl-11-keto-beta-boswellic acid (AKBA) but a combination of dozens of them.

This book is addressing these issues under a rigorous medical perspective. There is no shortage of books on medicinal plants written by photochemists, but there is a shortage of books written by clinicians with hands-on experience in the use of plant extracts.

Pharma-standard (PS) supplements

"Dietary" supplements are the most commonly used of all complementary and alternative treatments. The meaning of alternative and complementary is misleading. Medicine is medicine, and these products are well within the boundaries of medicine. The two adjectives have been often used and are still used by big pharma operators to decrease their possible value and image in comparison with "patented" products.

Pharma-standard (PS) supplements are generally safe and widely available — usually without prescription — and can usually be obtained without consulting a physician. However, the first indication for the use of supplements should be based on clinical grounds and upon the suggestions of a physician.

The Food and Drug Administration (FDA) regulates supplements differently from drugs. Quality control and good manufacturing processes are monitored, but the FDA does not define or ensure standardization of the active ingredients or their efficacy. Safety is always considered as the first issue, and most supplements available in the market can be defined as safe.

Definition

The Dietary Supplement Health Education Act (DSHEA) 1994 defines a dietary supplement as "any product (excluding tobacco and its derivatives) — in pill, capsule, tablet or liquid form — containing vitamins, mineral, herb or other product derived from plants, amino acid or other known dietary substance that is intended as a supplement to the normal diet". Certain hormones, such as dehydroepiandrosterone (DHEA), a precursor to androgens and estrogens, and melatonin, are regulated as dietary supplements and not as prescription drugs.

Labeling

The DSHEA requires that the product label clearly identify the product as a dietary supplement and notify the consumer that the suggested "claims" for the supplement have not been evaluated by the FDA. The label usually lists the ingredients, indicating them by name, indicating their quantity and total weight and must identify plant elements from which the ingredients are derived. Manufacturers are permitted to make claims about the product's structure and function (e.g., good for urinary tract health) but cannot make or imply specific claims for the product as it is not considered a drug and cannot be considered a specific therapy (e.g., treats UTIs).

Safety and efficacy

Dietary supplements (defined as "supplements") are generally safe and may be considered good for health problems. Supplements are considered effective for treating specific risk conditions or preclinical and even clinical conditions. Most supplements are natural (i.e., derived from plants) and often their history is supported by centuries of use in traditional systems of medicine. The FDA does not require manufacturers of supplements to prove their complete safety (i.e., in case of interactions with drugs) or efficacy (although generally, supplements must have a long history of safety). Usually the extraction of the supplements from plants or other sources should be without chemical or solvents that may interfere with the structure and potential toxicity of the products.

Most supplements have not been studied in a clinical atmosphere under big pharma rules and conditions. Most supplements are unpatented and their low income (relative to big pharma products) usually means that formal clinical study of a PS supplement would be extremely expensive considering the revenues of the product. Evidence suggesting safety or efficacy of most supplements comes from some case reports. Manufacturers and distributors of supplements must still report serious adverse events and tolerability problems to the FDA through the MedWatch system.

Some supplements (e.g., FO, chondroitin–glucosamine, saw palmetto) have now proved to be safe and useful complements to standard medical managements and therapy and can be considered models. Evidence concerning the safety and efficacy of supplements is increasing. More and more clinical studies are being completed, most of which are available at the National Institutes of Health's National Center for Complementary and Alternative Medicine (NCCAM) website (www.nccam.nih.gov/research/clinicaltrials). Most important papers are published in peer-review journals and quoted in Medline or Pubmed and important databases. However, each PS supplement formulation is different from another.

Studies which are valid for one product cannot be applied to all products derived from the same source. Here we are considering PS supplements that at least within a specific product formulation have constant, defined standards, dosages and preventive or therapeutic schemes, clearly defined by previous clinical/supplement studies.

Purity and standardization

Limited regulation means that supplements are not monitored to ensure the amount of active ingredients claimed by the manufacturers. Most producers do however monitor the quantity and quality of their products. The supplement must be carefully produced and tested to ensure it does not contain unlisted ingredients which may be inert or even harmful (e.g., natural toxins, bacteria, pesticides, lead or other heavy metals).

Supplements may also contain variable amounts of active ingredients, especially when whole plant-derived products are ground or made into extracts. However this is a "moral" issue, for the producer and most high-quality products, e.g., when different extracts from different years are blended, may always keep the same standards within very narrow limits. It is the responsibility of the user to carefully consider the quality of the products s/he uses and its standards; otherwise, consumers may put themselves at risk of receiving less, more or in some cases, none of the active ingredients.

Most plant-derived supplements include several complex compounds and substances. The most active or effective ingredient is not always known. A lack of standardization (which does not happen with high-quality products that we define as "pharma standard") means that not only may products vary from different producers or manufacturers but also that different batches produced by the same manufacturer may differ. Product variability is a constant source of problems and the conduct of rigorous scientific trials and comparison of results among different trials becomes difficult. However, supplements that have been standardized at pharma level may include indications explaining the type of standardization on the label to help consumers make "informed" choices.

Regulations governing the production and marketing of supplements in the US include rules for Good Manufacturing Practices (GMPs) that improve and strengthen standards for cleanliness of manufacturing facilities and equipment, as well as the purity (lack of contamination) of raw materials. GMPs also ensure proper labeling, packaging and storage of the finished product.

Other improvements in supplements and their use

The other improvements are as follows:

1. Additional areas of improvements of the use of PS supplement applications in preventive and clinical medical applications may include the following:
   a. Definition of the correct use of PS supplements instead of conventional drugs (i.e., in periods of remission, a supplement could be used instead of more expensive standard drug treatments which may cause more side effects and may be interactive with other treatments used concomitantly).
   b. Stability of PS supplements (particularly those derived from *vegetalia*) once manufactured. Specific blending procedure may be needed. The quantity and relative compositions of elements in a plant extract are variable every year due to rain, sun and climatic factors.
2. To keep a reasonable standard that includes defined ranges of the active compounds, appropriate blending (including compounds from several different years) is usually needed. This is a major skill in the preparation of PS supplements.
3. Possible toxicity as a single product and in connection with other treatments.
4. Relative toxicity considering special situations (i.e., renal or heart failure) should also be considered.
5. The possible (positive or negative) interactions between PS supplements and "standard" drugs should be defined for different types of patient and clinical situations.

At the moment, most information about significant interactions or negative effects derives from experience with sporadic, individual reports and some referenced case reports. However, many physicians, healthcare operators and patients believe and have experienced the benefit of nonstandard and PS supplements. Patients (and subjects with a risk condition) often use supplements with or without their physician's suggestion or knowledge. In some cases, patients may not inform physicians if they use supplements or may conceal their use for several reasons. Therefore any clinical outpatient history should specifically, clearly and periodically include *explicit questions about the use of supplements* (including queries regarding complementary or alternative therapies, including dietary and nutritional supplements).

Most physicians include some supplement use into their management and practice. Reasons include proven benefit of the supplement, a need to control the use of "standard drug treatments", the desire to ensure that supplements are used safely by patients (who may use supplements anyway) and according to defined safety rules. Also many physicians believe (according to scientific considerations and experience) that supplements (particularly PS supplements) are safe and effective.

There are limited results and information to guide patients when considering safety. Many patients might incorrectly assume that a "safe" product may be overdosed or used too often without problems. Overall, the number of problems due to dietary and PS supplements is generally less in comparison with drugs when considering the number of doses taken. The supplement, if correctly manufactured and used — according to rules in the right conditions — is generally safe.

Quality is essential

It is important to purchase all PS supplements from a well-known, high-quality producer. For example, it is considered recommended to buy supplements made in Germany or in Switzerland because in these countries they are generally regulated as drugs, and thus the preparations and standards are superior, much stricter than those of the US or in the Far East. Generally, low cost, bad packaging, lack of precise information about the compounds and lack of clear instructions indicate bad quality.

2

Common PS Supplements

The following supplements are widely used and are popular, generally considered effective, and have a list of medical references and particularly indications about their safety.

Beanblock

This is a dry extract of *Phaseolus vulgaris* characterized by a standardized composition in alpha amylase inhibitor, with inhibiting activity of 1,400 units/mg and phytohaemagglutinin (haemagglutinating activity equal to 15 haemagglutinating units/mg). This PS supplement has shown efficacy in controlling weight in overweight subjects, otherwise healthy individuals, and in helping in different overeating models. It could be a natural alternative or a supplementary measure to other weight control products. Beanblock can be generally used as an appetite regulator (but appetite is difficult to quantify) and a "control system" to decrease sugar and high-calorie-food absorption. No significant side effects have been observed. New studies are in progress.

Black cohosh (*Actaea racemosa*)

Black cohosh is the underground stem of a plant. Native Americans used black cohosh to treat gynecological and other disorders, including sore throats, kidney problems, and depression. The extract is standardized to contain a well-defined quantity of triterpenes. Black cohosh does not contain significant amounts of phytoestrogens that can explain its estrogen-like effects, but it contains small amounts of anti-inflammatory compounds, including salicylic acid (Figure 1).

PS supplements of black cohosh are considered useful for menopausal symptoms (hot flushes, mood changes, tachycardia, vaginal dryness), for some menstrual symptoms, and they have been used for joint pain, arthralgias in rheumatoid arthritis (RA) or osteoarthritis (OA). Evidence regarding benefits in controlling menstrual symptoms is conflicting but effects may be very individual. Patients may try the supplement, and if they find a benefit, they may avoid more complex, prescription drugs that may produce some side effects.

A recent meta-analysis (but this type of evaluation is very inconclusive for supplements from different producers) supports these claims. Study design, clinical targets, dosages and pharmaceutical characteristics of black cohosh preparations define clinical outcomes. Some recent investigations with PS supplements have indicated that these supplements have some beneficial effects on the physiological pathways underlying age-related disorders like osteoporosis. Some other recent findings suggest that a part of the clinically relevant effects of black cohosh supplement may be due to compounds that bind and activate serotonin receptors.

A derivate from serotonin with high affinity to serotonin receptors (*N*-methylserotonin) has been identified in black cohosh. Other complex molecules (triterpene glycosides, cycloartanes) have been shown to reduce cytokine-induced bone loss (osteoporosis) by blocking osteoclastogenesis. 23-*O*-acetylshengmanol-3-*O*-β-D-xylopyranoside, a cycloartane glycoside from *Actaea racemosa*, has been identified as a modulator of gamma-aminobutyric acid (GABA) receptors with sedative activity.

Adverse effects are uncommon (headache and gastrointestinal (GI) problems). Dizziness, diaphoresis and hypotension (only with high dosages) have been reported. PS supplements from black cohosh do not interfere with any drugs as far as we know. Theoretically, black cohosh supplements are contraindicated in patients with aspirin intolerance, liver disease, hormone-sensitive cancers (breast cancer), stroke, or high BP. The *US Pharmacopeia* (USP) recommends that black cohosh supplements

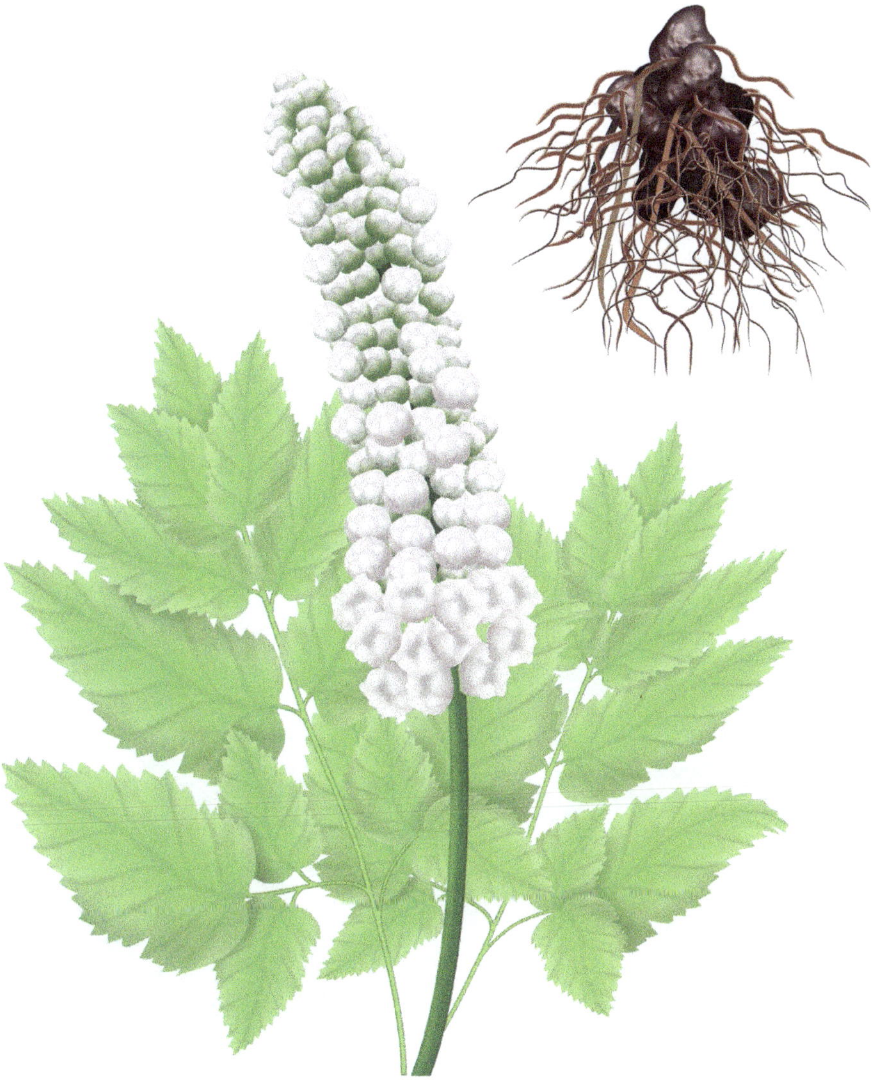

Figure 1: Black cohosh.

should be labeled with a warning declaring that they may be hepatotoxic. Long-term use of black cohosh may cause thickening of the womb possibly leading to an increased risk of womb cancer. Studies on women using black cohosh preparations did not detect estrogenic effects on the breast.

Boswellia

Boswellia serrata has a long history of medicinal use and has been developed for many applications, including topical use. PS supplements from *Boswellia serrata* include boswellic acid and other pentacyclic triterpene acids. Beta-boswellic acid is considered the major constituent in the extract and supplements. *Boswellia* supplements decrease polymorphonuclear leukocyte infiltration and migration, modulate or decrease antibody synthesis and the anticorpal response. The extract almost totally inhibits the classical complement pathway (Figure 2).

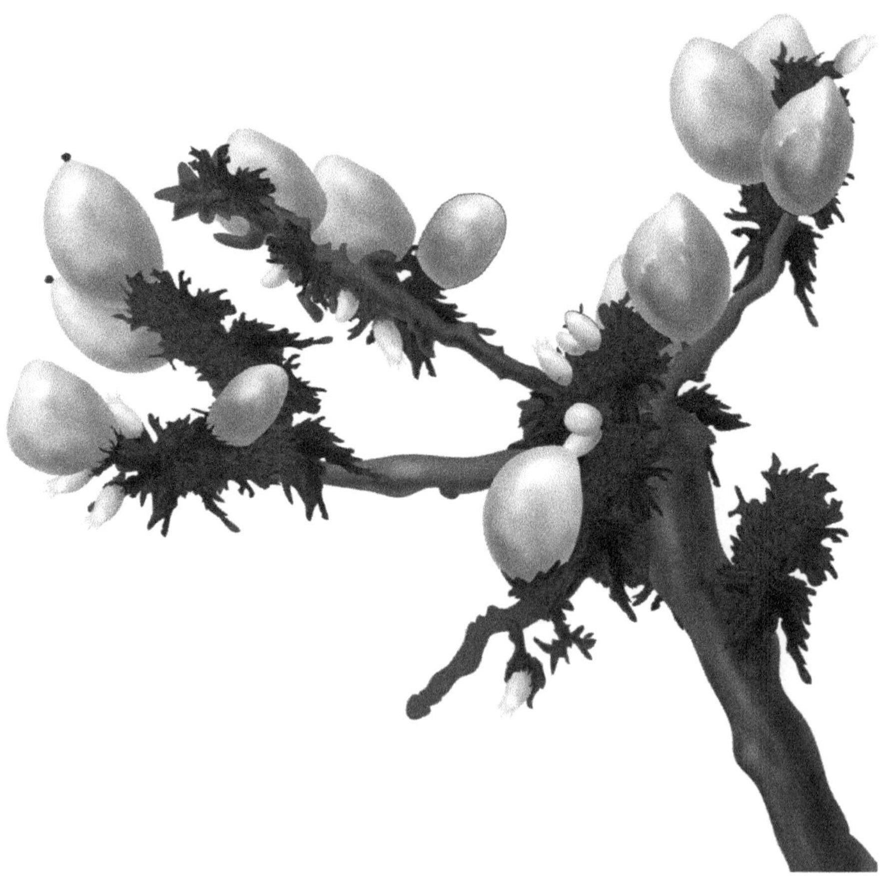

Figure 2: *Boswellia* plant.

PS supplements of *Boswellia* have a potent analgesic and anti-inflammatory activity that controls and reduces pain and inflammation of joints in patients with arthrosis. *Boswellia* PS supplements and *Boswellia* extracts have been used for the primary or supplementary management of OA and several other inflammatory conditions with significant clinical results. In these studies, even with different dosages and preparations, *Boswellia* has shown a very good level of tolerability and safety.

A recent *Boswellia* preparation (a standardized phytoextract from the bark of *Boswellia serrata*) includes essential oils from boswellic acid. The standardization process ensures higher bioavailability and efficacy. Its anti-inflammatory efficacy is broadly comparable to non-steroidal anti-inflammatory drugs (NSAIDs). *Boswellia* extracts inhibit some proin-flammatory mediators such as S-lipoxygenase and leukotrienes.

New, purified PS supplements and extracts of *Boswellia* do not cause side effects particularly GI ulcerative complications and are more active in comparison with other previously available *Boswellia* products. The effects of *Boswellia* supplements and preparations appear to persist longer (particularly in subjects with significant knee degeneration) and appear to be more effective than other products used to manage OA (i.e., chondroitin or glucosamine). The supplement seems to act rapidly and in a larger and wider number of patients.

This compound can now be considered an important effective supplementary treatment in OA patients, particularly in the "remission" phases or when signs/symptoms are reduced or minimal. *Boswellia* PS supplements are also very safe (large safety studies are in progress) and can be specifically used for self-medication. Other applications showing positive effects of *Boswellia* PS supplements include the improvement of deteriorated cognitive function (very difficult to evaluate), some chronic inflammatory diseases (rheumatoid arthritis, bronchial asthma, ulcerative colitis, Crohn's disease) (Figure 3).

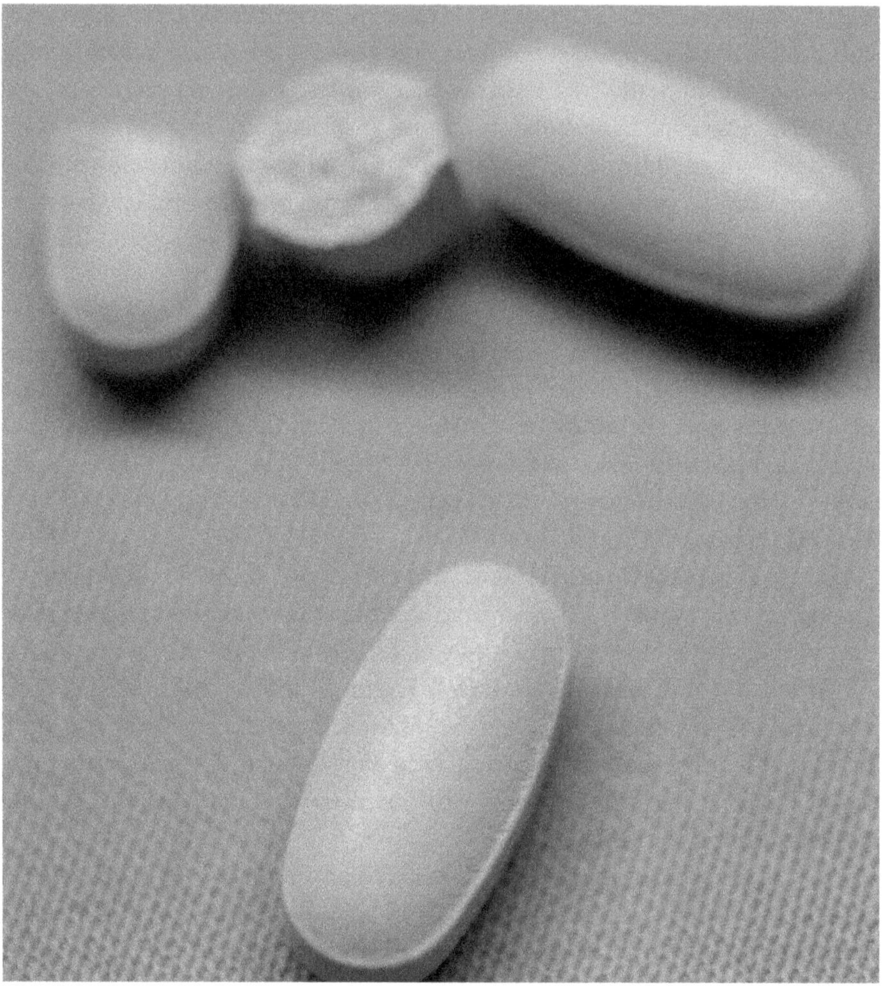

Figure 3: *Boswellia* pills.

Centella asiatica

Centella asiatica (CA) (formerly known as *Hydrocotyle asiatica*, also known as *Centella asiatica o Gotu kola*), is a member of the parsley family. It is native to India, Madagascar, Sri Lanka, Africa, Australia, China and Indonesia. CA is a small, herbaceous, annual plant of the family Mackinlayaceae or subfamily Mackinlayoideae of family Apiaceae. CA has a long history of use. It has been used medicinally since 2000 AD even to treat leprosy, to

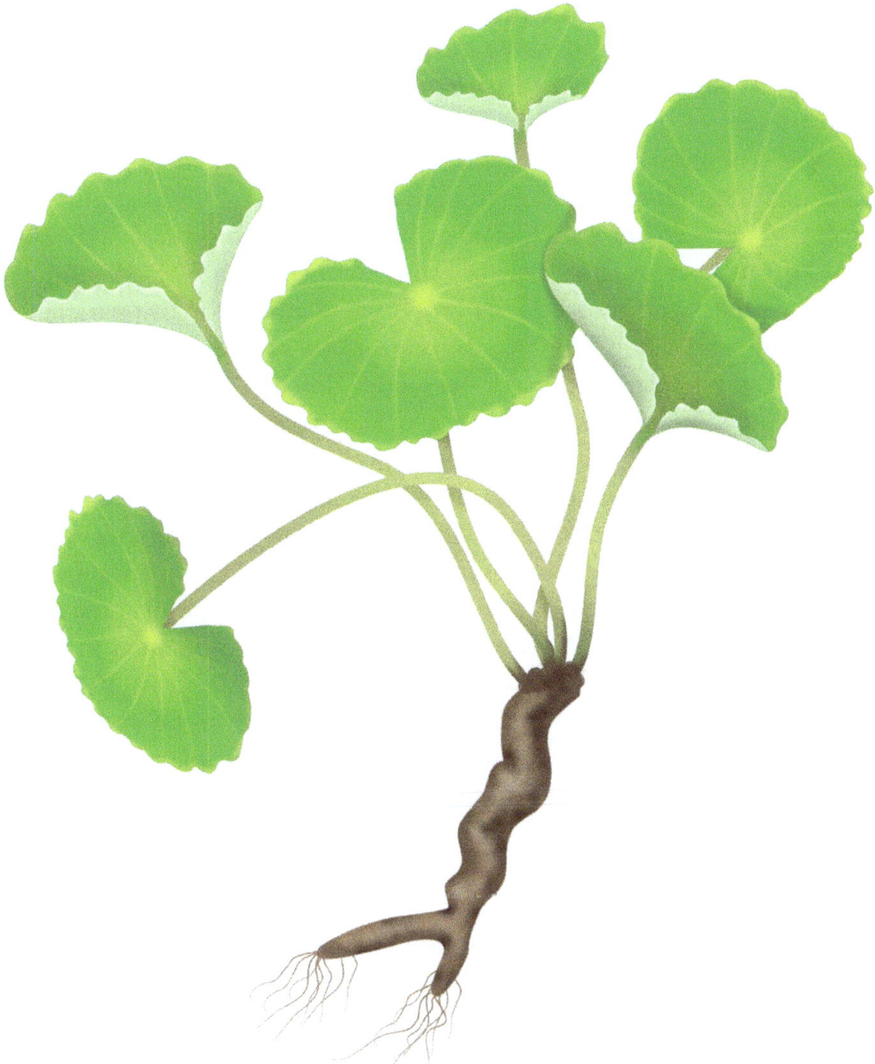

Figure 4: *Centella asiatica.*

treat wounds and gonorrhea and to treat fever and respiratory infections in China (Figure 4).

CA has large amounts of pentacyclic triterpenoids including asiaticoside, brahmoside, asiatic acid, and brahmic acid also known as madecassic acid. Other products include centellose, centelloside, and madecassoside. The most common use of CA in PS supplements in the US is in the supplementary treatment for varicose veins (VV) and chronic venous insufficiency (CVI).

Several studies using total triterpenic fraction of CA (TTFCA) in the management of CVI with leg swelling, VV, pain, itching, atrophic skin changes and ulcers and in patients with postthrombotic limbs have indicated significant improvements in signs and symptoms. CVI has also been evaluated in several prolonged studies, also involving the microcirculation. Results from these microcirculatory studies suggest that TTFCA produces moderate but significant benefits on objective and subjective parameters associated with CVI. TTFCA also appears to promote wound healing (venous ulcers) possibly through the modulation and stimulation of collagen synthesis. New products, now available, replicate the same effects.

The modulation of collagen is an important aspect of *Centella* and PS CA supplement. Too much collagen causes cheloids after burns, particularly in children, and causes an abnormal growth in venous ulcerations leading to irregular scarring and delayed healing. Finally an abnormal accumulation of collagen causes the irregular growth and progression of atherosclerotic plaques. A recent, long-term clinical evaluation indicates that the use of TTFCA (in association with Pycnogenol®) is effective in modulating the growth of atherosclerotic plaques in carotid and femoral arteries. Independent of the control of risk factors, the plaques grow less and slower and plaque progression is generally delayed.

Safety

The FDA does not strictly regulate CA as the other supplements. Theoretically, CA may cause an increase in drowsiness caused by sedatives (i.e., benzodiazepines such as lorazepam, barbiturates, codeine) and interact with alcohol. Caution is advised when driving or using machinery.

Side effects

Minor effects can be observed including stomach upset and nausea. *Centella* grows along ditches and in low, wet areas. The plant frequently suffers from high levels of bacterial and metal contamination, possibly from having been harvested from sewage ditches or close to contaminated water. Because the plant is aquatic, it is especially sensitive to pollutants in the water, which are easily incorporated into the plant. Apparently, the plant produced in Madagascar is more effective (and cleaner) than comparable plants from other regions particularly in modulating collagen.

Chamomile

The flower of chamomile is dried and used in infusion as a tea or used topically as a simple extract (Figure 5).

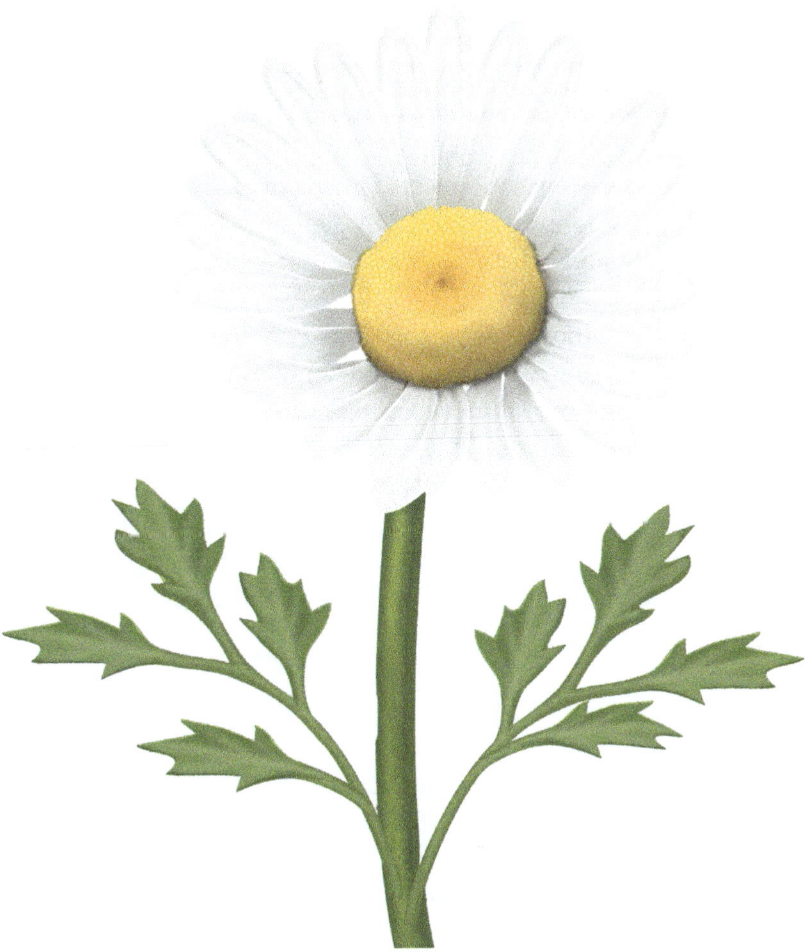

Figure 5: Chamomile.

Claims

Chamomile may reduce fever and inflammation, act as a mild sedative, may relieve stomach cramps and indigestion and may promote healing of gastric ulcers. An essential oil containing bisabolol is the main constituent. Chamomile may increase the effects of anticoagulants and sedatives (including alcohol) and could decrease the absorption of iron supplements. PS supplements are difficult to find. Most uses include the full flower extract.

Coenzyme Q10 (CoQ10)

Coenzyme Q10 (CoQ10) (ubiquinone) is a powerful and common antioxidant and a cofactor for mitochondrial ATP generation. The reduced form of CoQ10 regenerates vitamin E from the α-tocopheroxyl radical, interfering with the propagation step. During oxidative stress, interaction of H_2O_2 with metal ions bound to DNA generates hydroxyl radicals, and CoQ10 efficiently prevents the oxidation of bases, particularly, in mitochondrial DNA.

In contrast to other antioxidants, this compound inhibits both the initiation and the propagation of lipid and protein oxidation. It also regenerates other antioxidants such as vitamin E. The circulating CoQ10 in LDL prevents oxidation of LDL, which may provide benefit in cardiovascular diseases. The levels of CoQ10 are lower in older people, in people with chronic diseases (i.e., chronic cardiac problems, cancer, Parkinson's disease, diabetes, HIV/AIDS and muscular dystrophies) and in patients using statins. It is not clear how low levels contribute to these disorders.

Claims

CoQ10 is considered to be useful because of its antioxidant effect and role in energy metabolism. Specific claims include an anticancer effect mediated by immune stimulation, decreased insulin requirements in patients with diabetes, slowed progression of Parkinson's disease, efficacy in treatment of heart failure, and protection against some types of cardiotoxicity. Although some preliminary studies suggest CoQ10 may be useful in improving or cotreating these disorders, results are not clear and more studies are needed.

Adverse effects

CoQ10 may decrease response to warfarin. There are case reports of GI symptoms (including loss of appetite, abdominal pain, nausea, vomiting) and neurological central nervous system (CNS) symptoms (dizziness, headache, tinnitus, photophobia, irritability). Other adverse effects include itching, rash, fatigue and flu-like symptoms. CoQ10 is not generally indicated for people who exercise vigorously. The common use of statins to treat high lipids in atherosclerosis is known to reduce the levels of CoQ10, and may even be responsible for causing heart failure. Supplementation with CoQ10 supplements may restore the levels of CoQ10.

Inhibition of CoQ10 by statins and beta blockers

CoQ10 shares a biosynthetic pathway with cholesterol. The synthesis of an intermediary precursor of CoQ10, mevalonate, is inhibited by some beta blockers, blood-pressure drugs and by statins (cholesterol-lowering drugs). Statins can reduce serum levels of CoQ10 by up to 40%. Supplementation with CoQ10 may be considered in any treatment that may reduce endogenous production of CoQ10.

Colostrum

Colostrum is a milky fluid that comes from the breasts of humans, cows, and other mammals the first few days after giving birth, before true milk appears. It contains proteins, carbohydrates, fats, vitamins, minerals, and proteins (antibodies) that fight disease-causing agents such as bacteria and viruses. Antibody levels in colostrums can be 100 times higher than levels in regular cow's milk. Colostrum is a GI tract antioxidant and an important aid in the prevention and treatment of problems linked to asthenia, lack of appetite, anemia, pathological conditions, convalescence and metabolic disorders. Colostrum is the first type of milk — rich in immunoglobulins — produced by the mother's breast after childbirth.

Colostrum initially nourishes the newborn for the first few days of life and at the same time protects the child from the potential aggression of the outside environment at a moment of great vulnerability for the organism. The intestinal contact surface is a very large possible site of lethal contamination in babies before they have the protective effect of their immunoglobulins. Colostrum is considered as the "baby's first vaccination" considering the large number of antibodies it contains.

Among the most vulnerable parts of the newborns, the GI tract is very vulnerable the days after birth. The vulnerability does not disappear after the first few days of life and may lead to several problems and disorders, sometimes limited to unpleasant symptoms and sometimes leading to acute or chronic diseases. A large number of diseases have origins in the intestinal tract. The term "intestinal dysbiosis" has been created to identify a condition of reduced intestinal defensive function with immunologic, inflammatory and infectious problems. Colostrum restores the GI environment and as a consequence, systemic health not only in newborns but also in adults.

Proline-rich polypeptides (PRPs) have been discovered in colostrum (they are present in blood plasma). These polypeptides have been named colostrinins (CLNs), transfer factors or PRPs. They function as signal-transducing molecules that have the unique effect of modulating the immune system, turning it up when the body comes under attack from pathogens or other disease agents and damping it when the danger is eliminated or neutralized.

At first thought to transfer immunity from one immune system to another, it now appears that PRP simply stimulates cell-mediated immunity. PS colostrum has been used to prevent infective and viral episodes. A recent study indicated that colostrum as a PS supplement can be used for the prevention of flu and cold in otherwise healthy subjects. Colostrum was superior (in preventing viral and flu episodes) to flu vaccination both in healthy and high-risk cardiovascular subjects and subjects with pulmonary disease. Colostrum was also useful to prevent a number of hospital admissions and moderate to severe complications in older subjects. Colostrum is indicated in improving weakness (i.e., after convalescence) in elderly people to prevent flu and infections and in weaker people. It has also been used and abused by athletes. Bovine colostrum is **not** on the banned drug list of the International Olympic Committee.

Adverse effects

No significant side effects have been reported. A subject allergic to cow's milk or milk products may also be allergic to bovine colostrum. In this condition, it is best to avoid colostrum supplementation.

Chondroitin sulfate

Chondroitin sulfate (CS) is a glycosaminoglycan, an essential and natural component of any cartilage. It is generally extracted from shark or cow cartilage; it can be manufactured synthetically. It is often combined with glucosamine. CS is used to manage OA and its signs/symptoms. In combination with glucosamine, CS reduces joint pain and improves joint mobility; these effects allow a significant reduction of the doses of conventional anti-inflammatory drugs. Effects on symptoms are seen after 6–24 months of treatment. Structural effects on the joints are seen over longer periods but appear unclear. The dose is generally around 600 mg (per os) once daily or 400 mg, three times daily.

Adverse effects

No serious adverse effects have been seen considering that products including CS are widely used by a large number of patients for long periods. Common adverse effects are stomach pain, nausea and GI symptoms. CS may affect the activity of the anticoagulant warfarin. PS products including CS are generally safe, but people with asthma, blood-clotting disorders, or prostate cancer should use some caution when taking it or consider alternatives.

Cranberry

In Britain, cranberry may refer to the native species *Vaccinium oxycoccos*, while in North America, cranberry may refer to *Vaccinium macrocarpon*. Cranberries are fruits that are consumed whole, made into food products (jellies, juices) extracts and PS supplements (Figure 6).

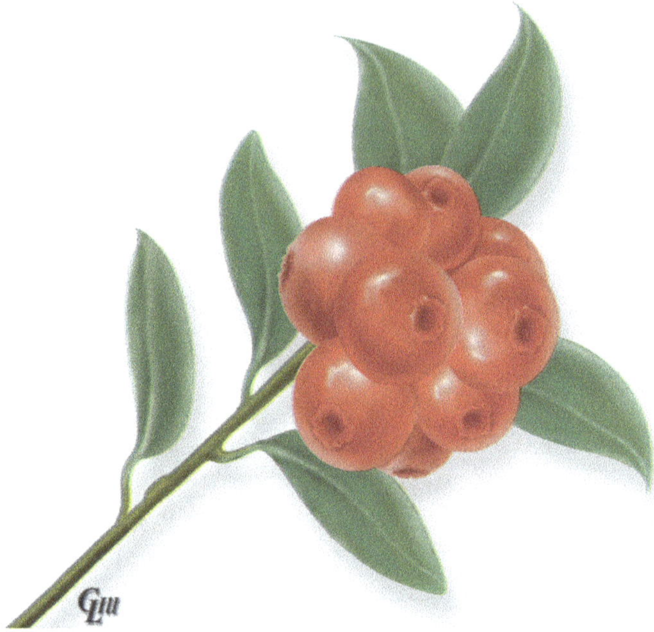

(a)

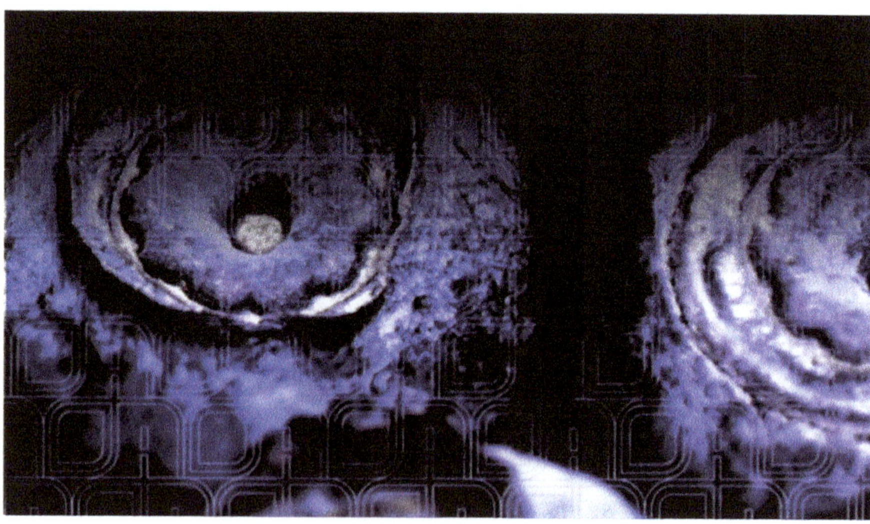

(b)

Figure 6: (a) Cranberry plant and (b) cranberry.

Claims

PS cranberry supplements help to prevent and relieve the symptoms of urinary tract infections (UTIs) and postinfection inflammation. The efficacy of cranberries in preventing UTIs has been shown in several studies. Natural unprocessed cranberry juice contains anthocyanidins which prevent *Escherichia coli* from colonizing the urinary tract wall. Cranberry juice may reduce fever in some patients.

Problems may arise with the lack of validation of a standard method for the quantification of A-type proanthocyanidins. In the case of most cranberry extracts, it can be performed using several existing methods including, e.g., the *European Pharmacopoeia* method, liquid chromatography–mass spectrometry (LC–MS) or a modified 4-dimethyl-aminocinnamaldehyde (DMAC) colorimetric method. This may lead to difficulties in evaluating the real quality of extracts from different origins.

Studies indicate that quality varies greatly from one commercial cranberry product to another. PS supplements are becoming more common and are being produced with defined quantity of active substances. Recent studies in different types of patients indicate that a cranberry PS supplement decreases the number of urinary infection episodes in 2 months in the following cases:

1. prone subjects,
2. elder patients with prostatic hypertrophy,
3. younger subjects.

Good results have been obtained in premenopausal women in several studies.

Adverse effects

No adverse effects are known. However, because most cranberry juices include sugar to offset its tart taste, diabetics should use cranberry juice with caution and with artificial sweeteners. This problem is overcome by PS supplements in capsules. Cranberry supplements increase urinary acidity and, theoretically, may promote stone formation in patients with story of uric acid kidney stones. Cranberry supplementation may occasionally increase the effects of warfarin.

Creatine

Phosphocreatine is stored in muscle. This compound donates phosphate to ADP and rapidly replenishes ATP during anaerobic muscle contraction. It is synthesized endogenously in the liver from arginine, glycine and methionine. Creatine is found in milk, meat and some fish. Creatine may improve physical and athletic performance also reducing muscular fatigue. Creatine has been found effective at increasing the efficiency of exercise in short maximal efforts (sprinting, weightlifting). It has a defined therapeutic use in muscle phosphorylase deficiency (glycogen storage disease type V or McArdle disease) and gyrate atrophy of the choroid and retina. Some studies indicate possible effects in Parkinson's disease and amyotrophic lateral sclerosis.

Adverse effects

Creatine may cause weight gain (possibly because of an increase in muscle mass) and increases in serum creatinine. Minor GI symptoms, dehydration, electrolytic imbalance, and muscle cramps have been reported.

Curcumin

Curcumin is the yellow pigment of turmeric (*Curcuma longa* L.), the most popular spice in Indian cuisine and a major ingredient of curry (Figure 7). The dietary intake of curcumin in Asian countries can reach much as 200 mg/d. In the UK population, the mean and maximum reported use levels of curcumin have been estimated, combining the use of curcumin from naturally occurring curcumin in foods (turmeric as a spice and in curry powder) and from its use as a food color, at over 50 mg/d and 210 mg/d, respectively, in the adult population. Turmeric has a long history of medicinal use in India to control or treat many conditions.

Cellular studies on curcumin have validated most of its traditional uses and have indicated its potential to control some risk conditions and

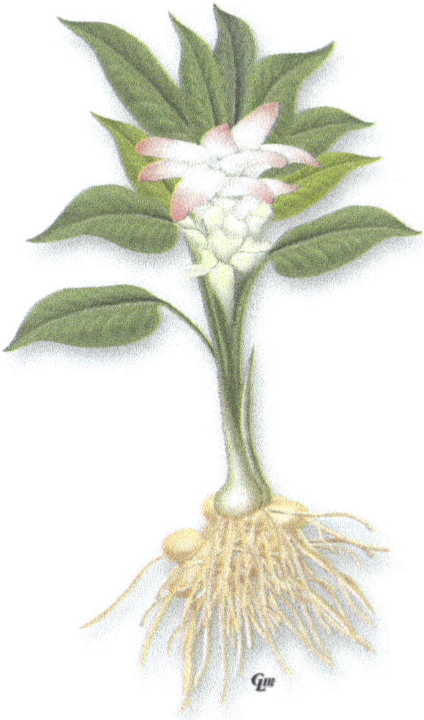

Figure 7: Curcumin plant.

diseases. With some 4,000 preclinical investigations, curcumin is one of the best studied and known natural products within the biomedical literature. Curcumin has recently emerged as a significant, important compound to control and treat natural and abnormal inflammatory responses. Its actions include both a direct and a genomic activity on relevant enzymes, action on transcription factors and on cytokines. Recent clinical evidence has raised a great interest for curcumin, particularly considering the new PS formulations. Still, most of the beneficial effects of curcumin are shown or suggested by epidemiological studies. Animal models — as for most supplements — may be interesting but hardly conclusive.

The new PS supplement curcumin (Meriva®) as bioavailable curcumin is a patented delivery form. Curcumin and soy lecithin are formulated in a 1:2 weight ratio, and two parts of microcrystalline cellulose are then added to improve flowability, with an overall content of curcumin in the final product of around 20%. Meriva® is based on Phytosome® technology aimed to improve the bioavailability of compounds like polyphenolics and triterpenoid acids, which are normally characterized by poor solubility both in water and in organic solvents.

Curcumin, just like most PS dietary phenolics, is not very soluble in water or in oily solvents but shows polar groups that interact via hydrogen bonding and polar interactions with complementary groups, like the polar heads of phospholipids. Thus, soy lecithin has a highly polarized head, with the negative charge of a phosphate group and the positive charge of the choline ammonium group, and can complex a variety of poorly soluble phenolics, including curcumin. Phenolics such as curcumin, show a high affinity for biological membranes, and once complexed with phospholipids, they are embedded into a lipidic matrix that can capitalize on the rapid exchange of phospholipids between biological membranes and the extracellular fluids, shuttling it into biological membranes. This mechanism greatly increases its cellular capitation.

Studies on Meriva® (complexed curcumin) have addressed the natural and abnormal inflammatory response process. The use of Meriva® for bone health is based on the capacity of this compound to interrupt most inflammatory responses signaling and increases antioxidant levels. Evidence indicates that bone health is better supported by agents that modulate multiple cellular targets and that curcumin has a great potential for the management of these conditions.

Curcumin (Meriva®) has shown its efficacy in individuals with knee arthrosis. Their symptoms (evaluated by the Western Ontario and McMaster Universities Osteoarthritis Index (WOMAC) score), mobility (studied by walking performance on a treadmill) and the overall inflammatory response function (C-reactive protein) improved in 3 months using Meriva® at 1 g/d (in two doses). The treadmill, particularly, indicated a significant improvement in walking. Also, it was noted that subjects using Meriva® used less standard treatments and managements with an appropriate reduction in costs.

Studies on visual impairment also indicated a significant action of curcumin (Meriva®). Other studies showed the effects on microcirculation in diabetic microangiopathy, on the inflammatory response and a positive effect on subjects exercising in sports. Another important study indicated that curcumin — as Meriva® — was effective in decreasing

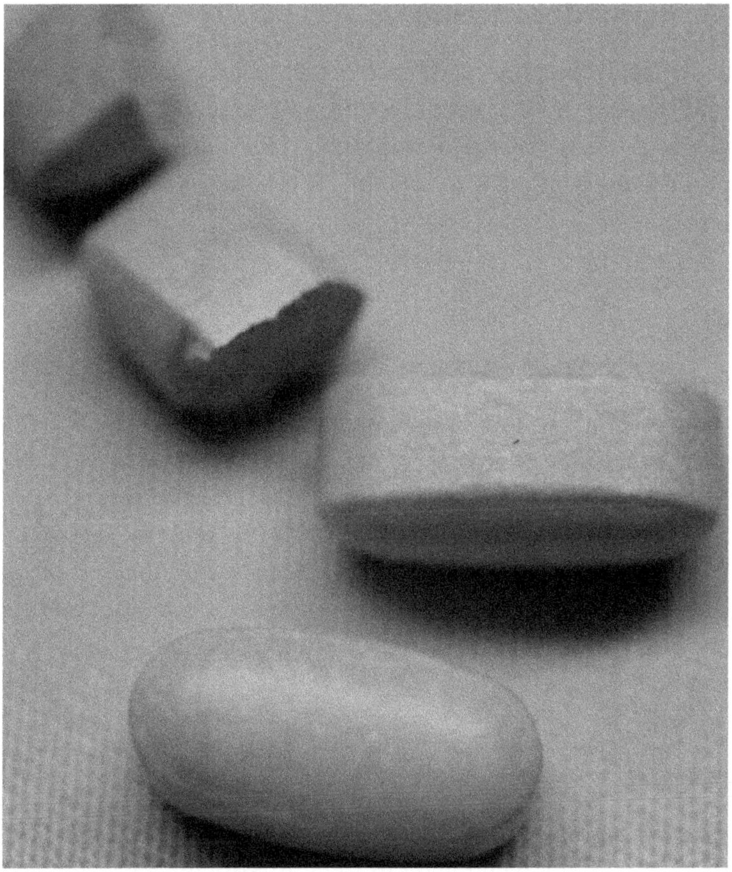

Figure 8: Curcumin pills.

unwanted, side effects, in subjects treated with radio and chemotherapy without changing the global effects of treatments.

Pharmacokinetics studies of curcumin include a broad range of experiences. In accordance with previous studies, 99% of curcumin — after oral administration — was present in plasma as glucuronides, with the remaining 1% being curcumin sulfate and free curcumin. Formulation with phospholipids led to a marked (over 20-fold) increase in the concentration of plasma curcumin (essentially glucuronides). Curcumin — in conclusion — is one of the most studied PS supplements and could be a model for other products' evaluation (Figure 8).

Dehydroepiandrosterone

Dehydroepiandrosterone (DHEA) is a steroid produced by the adrenal gland, precursor of estrogens and androgens. Effects on the body are similar to those of testosterone. DHEA can also be synthesized from precursors in the Mexican yam; this form is the most commonly available.

Claims

In women with adrenal insufficiency and in the healthy elderly subjects, there is very limited evidence to support the use of DHEA. DHEA supplements are said to improve mood, energy, sense of wellbeing, and the ability to perform better under stress. DHEA may also improve athletic performance, stimulate the immune system, deepen nightly sleep, lower cholesterol levels, decrease body fat, build muscles, reverse aging, improve brain function in patients with Alzheimer's disease and increase libido. Actually, the medicinal claims of DHEA are still unproven.

Adverse effects

Adverse effects are not well known and depend upon dosage. There are theoretical risks of gynecomastia in men, hirsutism in women and facilitation or stimulation of prostate and breast cancer. There are reports of mania and one of seizure, but it is quite possible that not all side effects have been reported.

DHEA supplements have been considered useful to improve memory functions in normal middle aged or older adults. DHEA has also been studied as a treatment for Alzheimer's disease, but at the moment, there is no evidence that the product may be effective. Studies also suggest that low serum levels of DHEA may be associated with coronary heart disease in men. At the moment, there is no evidence to indicate whether DHEA supplementation might have any significant cardiovascular action or benefit of the progression of the most common cardiovascular conditions. Some preliminary evidence indicates a short-term benefit of DHEA in patients with systemic lupus erythematosus. There is little evidence of long-term benefits or safety in these patients.

Echinacea

Originally, a North American wildflower, *Echinacea* contains a variety of biologically active substances. The *Echinacea* genus has nine species of flowers, commonly called *coneflowers. Echinacea purpurea* is most commonly used medicinally. The medicinal *Echinacea* products that are marketed and studied in clinical trials varied widely. They contain different species (*E. purpurea*, *E. angustifolia*, *E. pallida*), different organs (roots and herbs), different preparations (extracts and juice) and have different chemical compositions (Figure 9).

Studies are limited. The multiple meta-analyses are hopeless, as usual, comparing not apples with oranges but figs with meteorites, and as a result, these have no clinical meaning. The variability of the *Echinacea* products used in the several studies is impossibly large. The common cold may be affected by some *Echinacea* products. *Echinacea* may be used to stimulate the immune system. When taken at the start of a cold, it may shorten the duration of symptoms. Some topical preparations appear to promote wound healing.

Adverse effects

Adverse effects are usually mild and transitory (dizziness, fatigue, headache and GI symptoms). No other significant adverse effects are known. *Echinacea* should not be used in patients with autoimmune disorders, multiple sclerosis, AIDS, TB and after organ transplants, because it may stimulate T cells. However, the effects could be minimal and clinically irrelevant. *Echinacea* inhibits some cytochrome P-450 enzymes and stimulates others; it can therefore interact with some drugs metabolized by the same enzymes (anabolic steroids, azole antifungals, methotrexate). Some allergic reactions are possible in patients with pollen allergies.

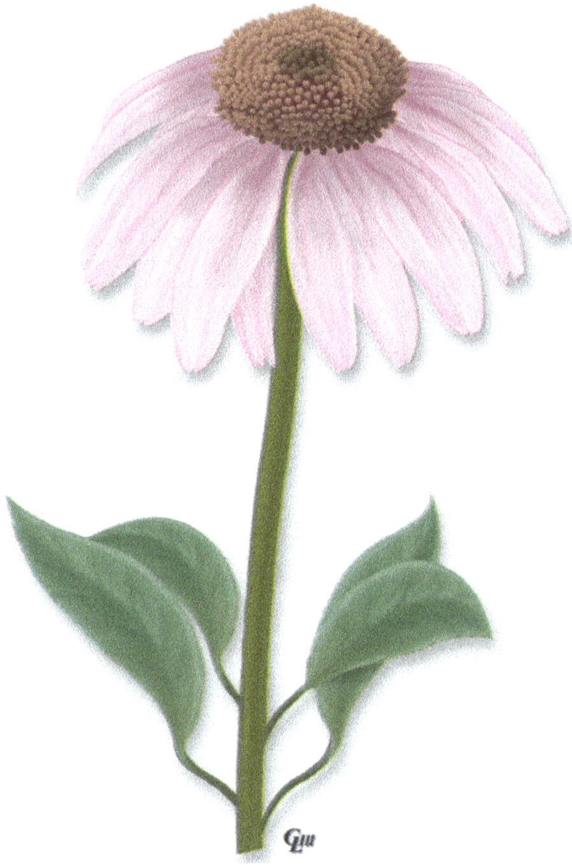

Figure 9: *Echinacea* plant.

Products containing *Echinacea* should not be used in children under the age of 12. Manufacturers label all oral *Echinacea* products that have product licenses for children with a warning that they should not be given to children under 12. As regards pregnancy, no study has yet found increased risk of birth defects associated with *Echinacea* during the first trimester, but pregnant women should avoid *Echinacea* products. As regards lactation, during breastfeeding, any product should be avoided, including all *Echinacea* products.

Among PS supplements, Immunoselect® (produced with *E. angustifolia* roots harvested in the US) is standardized to contain at least 4% of echinacoside, the major polyphenol in *E. angustifolia* root. It includes isobutylamides with anti-inflammatory and pain-relief action. *Echinacea purpurea* extract (≥0.8% of caftaric, chicoric, chlorogenic acids and echinacoside) is also a significant immunomodulator.

Polinacea® (also an immunomodulator from plants cultivated in Italy) is a standardized extract from the roots of *E. angustifolia*. These plants guarantee both a very high title on polysaccharide as well as any possible cross contamination between *Echinacea* species. The PS supplement contains a high-molecular-weight polysaccharide (IDN 5405) of around 20,000 Da identified for the very first time in the *E. angustifolia* root, specific of this plant that has been standardized to be devoid of isobutylamides (≤0.1%).

The standardization of the many products from the different plants is in progress. Without standards, the product is not clearly usable from a clinical point of view. *Echinacea* may also be very important as a cosupplement in other PS supplements.

Feverfew

Feverfew is a bushy perennial herb. The dried leaves are used in capsules, tablets and liquid extracts. Parthenolides and glycosides are thought to be the components responsible for its purported anti-inflammatory effects and relaxant effects on smooth muscle (Figure 10).

Claims

Feverfew is said to be effective in the prevention of migraine headaches. Evidence from three or four relatively small but well-designed studies supports these claims, but the largest and best designed of these studies does not. Differences among study findings may reflect the different formulations of feverfew used. Feverfew is also said to be useful for relieving menstrual pain, asthma and arthritis. *In vitro*, feverfew inhibits platelet aggregation.

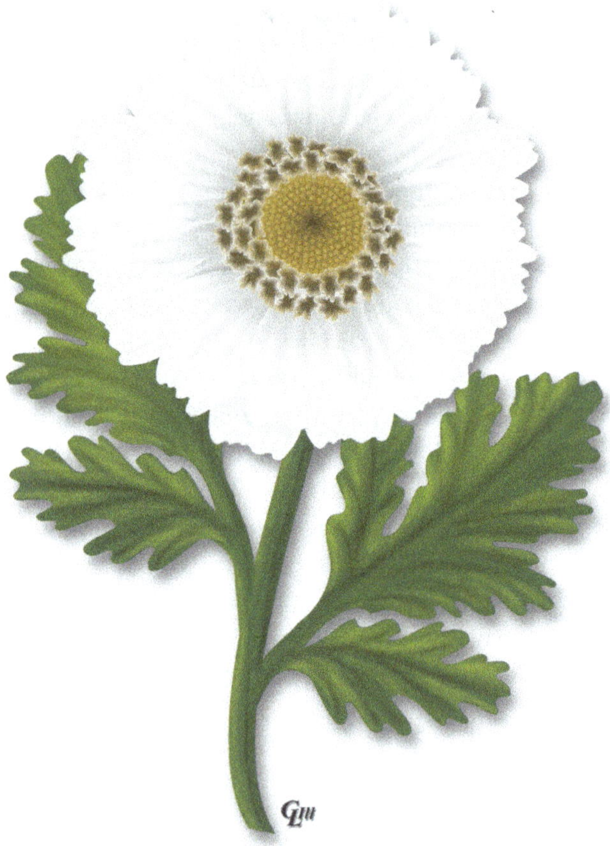

Figure 10: Feverfew.

Adverse effects

Mouth ulcers, contact dermatitis, dysgeusia, and mild GI symptoms have been described. Abrupt discontinuation may worsen migraines and cause nervousness and insomnia. Feverfew is contraindicated in pregnant women; in theory, it is contraindicated in patients taking other antimigraine drugs, iron supplements, nonsteroidal anti-inflammatory drugs (NSAIDs), antiplatelet drugs, or warfarin.

Fish oil

Fish oil (FO) is one of the best studied supplements. It is generally derived from the tissues of oily fish. FOs contain the omega-3 fatty acids eicosapentaenoic acid (EPA) and docosahexaenoic acid (DHA), precursors of certain eicosanoids that are known to reduce inflammation and have several other health benefits. FO may be extracted directly or concentrated and put in capsules to reach pharma standards. Active ingredients are omega-3 fatty acids (EPA and DHA). Western diets are typically low in omega-3 fatty acids.

Claims

FO supplementation is used for the prevention and treatment of atherosclerotic cardiovascular disease. There is a list of studies with strong scientific evidence suggesting that FO supplementation with EPA/DHA (from 80 to 1,500 mg daily) reduces the risk of myocardial infarction (MI) and death due to arrhythmia in patients with pre-existing coronary artery disease and using standard treatments.

FO also reduces triglycerides and its effects are dose dependent (25–40% with EPA/DHA 4 g/d); most PS supplements of FO slightly lower blood pressure (2–4 mmHg with EPA/DHA > 3 g/d). FO and omega-3 fatty acids have been studied in a variety of other conditions, such as depression, anxiety, oncological conditions, cancer (no clinical studies), retinal problems and macular degeneration. Benefits in these conditions need better evaluation in longer studies.

The effects of FO supplementation on prostate hypertrophy (cancer is out of the question) are not clear. There is a decreased risk with higher blood levels of EPA but an increased risk of more aggressive prostate cancer with higher blood levels of combined EPA and DHA. Some evidence of an association between high blood levels of omega-3 fatty acids and an increased cancer risk has been observed. However, cancer and PS supplements really have no connection. It is clear that prevention of any cancer may require long follow-up and large study populations.

Alzheimer's disease: A Cochrane meta-analysis (in June 2012) found no significant protective effect for cognitive decline for those aged 60 and over and who started taking fatty acids after this age. The analysis appears faulty (as most of these analyses, putting together different clinical conditions and different supplements) and suggests that there is no evidence that omega-3 fatty acid supplements provide a benefit for memory or concentration in later life. However, this kind of analysis is very questionable and there is not a PS supplement or a therapeutic or preventive protocol suitable for these conditions. This kind of analysis, often faulty with standard drugs and treatments is almost impossible for supplements that may have (and usually have) completely different standards and dosages.

Lupus: The disease activity, especially in the skin and joints, was reduced in patients who received FO supplements. There were also changes in platelets in patients who took the FO supplements. Inflammatory proteins were also reduced.

Psoriasis: Diets supplemented with cod oil have shown beneficial effects on some symptoms of psoriasis.

FO used during pregnancy may reduce an infant's sensitization to some food allergens, reducing frequency and severity of certain skin diseases in the first year of life. This effect may persist until adolescence with a reduction in prevalence or severity of eczema, hay fever and asthma.

Some national boards recommend a daily intake of 300–500 mg, while the US does not have recommendations for EPA and DHA. The American Heart Association recommends 250–500 mg/d of EPA and DHA. The FDA (US) recommends not exceeding 3 g/d of EPA and DHA omega-3 fatty acids, with no more than 2 g/d from a supplement. The concentrations of EPA and DHA in supplements can vary from between 8% and 80% of FO content. The concentration depends on the source of the omega-3s, how the oil is processed and the amounts of other ingredients included in the supplement.

Consumers of oily fish should be aware of the potential presence of heavy metals and fat-soluble pollutants like PCBs and dioxins, which are known to accumulate up the food chain. Generally, the benefits of fish intake far outweigh the potential risks. Microalgae oil is a vegetarian alternative to FO. Supplements produced from microalgae oil provide a balance of omega-3 fatty acids similar to FO, with a lower risk of pollutant exposure. Krill-derived FO is an important alternative and it is generally free of contaminants. Krill oil also contains naturally occurring astaxanthin, which has antioxidant activity and gives krill oil its natural red color.

Ginger

Ginger is extracted from the rhizome of the plant *Zingiber officinale* and consumed as a delicacy, medicine or spice. It derives its name to its genus and family (*Zingiberaceae*). Other notable members of this plant family are turmeric, cardamom and galangal. The distantly related dicots in the *Asarum* genus have the common name wild ginger because of their similar taste. The extracts are processed into dosed tablet form and PS supplements. Active ingredients include gingerols (which give ginger its flavor and odor) and shogaols (Figure 11).

Claims

Ginger is considered an antiemetic and antinausea, especially for nausea caused by motion sickness or pregnancy. It has been used to relieve intestinal cramps. Several studies indicate a beneficial effect in pregnancy-related nausea and vomiting. Ginger is also used as an anti-inflammatory and analgesic agent. It may have weak antibacterial properties and antiplatelet effects, but studies are limited or weak.

Ginger has a sialagogue action, stimulating the production of saliva, which makes swallowing easier. According to the American Cancer Society, ginger has been promoted as a cancer prevention tool, but there is no evidence in humans. A study at the University of Michigan has demonstrated that gingerols can inhibit growth of ovarian cancer cells *in vitro*. The clinical value of this finding is very relative. Ginger also affects arthritis pain and tends to lower lipids and cholesterol, but these effects have not been defined in large studies with PS supplements.

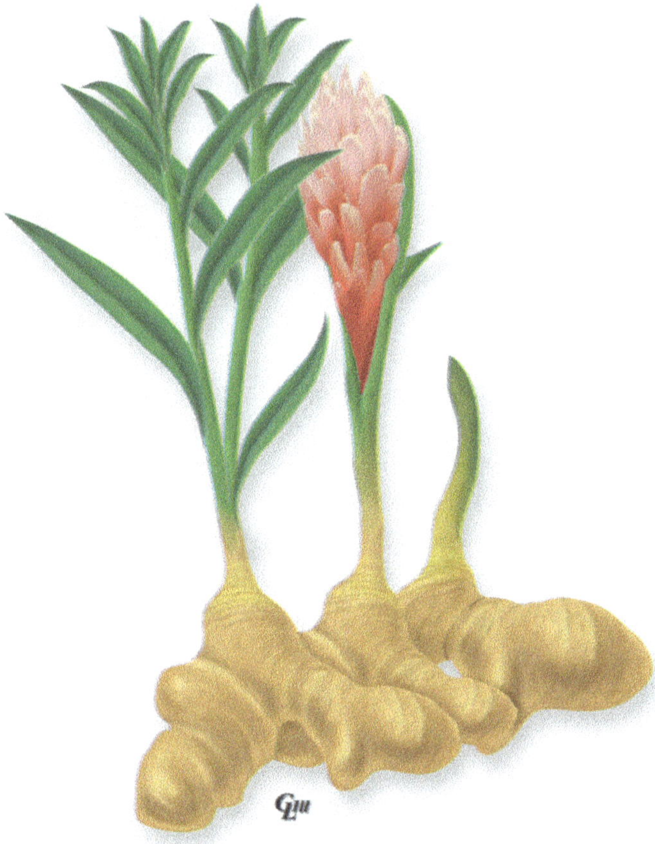

Figure 11: Ginger.

Adverse effects

Ginger is usually not harmful, but some people may have a burning sensation when they eat or drink the extracts (Figure 12). Nausea and dyspepsia have been reported. In theory, ginger should not be used in patients with bleeding or coagulation problems or treated with anticoagulants or antiplatelet drugs. Some reports also indicate that ginger may be mutagenic; therefore, the use in pregnant women should be limited, particularly in the first trimester.

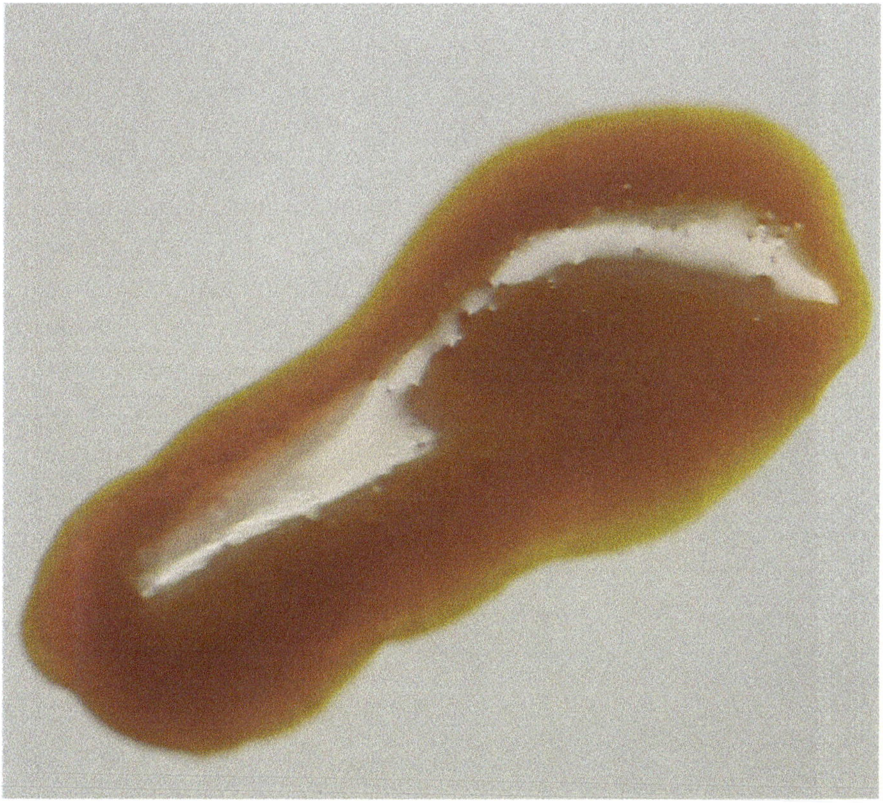

Figure 12: Ginger oil.

Ginkgo

Ginkgo biloba (GB) is prepared from the leaves of the ginkgo tree (commonly planted in the US for ornamental purposes). It is considered a fossil plant present in fossil from 270 million years. The plant is extremely resistant; some ginkgo trees survived the atomic blast in Hiroshima and are still alive (Figure 13).

Active ingredients are believed to be terpene ginkgolides and flavonoids. Extracts of ginkgo leaves contain flavonoid glycosides (myricetin and quercetin) and terpenoids (ginkgolides, bilobalides). The plant also contains biflavones; important constituents present in the leaves are the

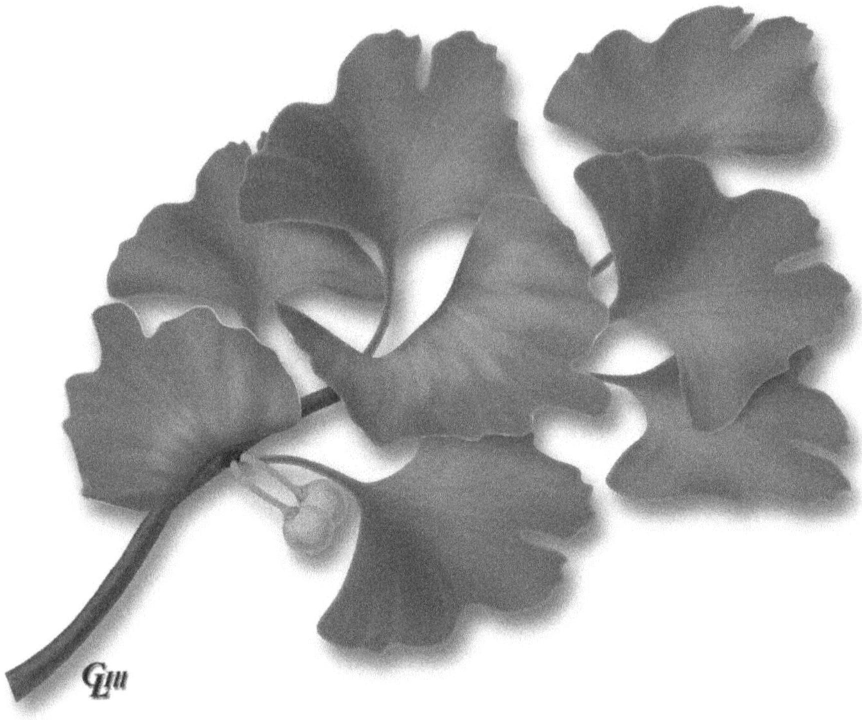

Figure 13: *Ginkgo biloba*.

terpene trilactones, i.e., ginkgolides A, B, C, J and bilobalide, many flavonol glycosides, biflavones, proanthocyanidins, alkylphenols, simple phenolic acids, 6-hydroxykynurenic acid, 4-*O*-methylpyridoxine and polyprenols.

The fruit of the ginkgo tree, which is quite malodorous, is not used in ginkgo products. Contact with the fruit pulp, which may be present under female ginkgo trees, can cause severe dermatitis. The raw seeds of the fruit are toxic and can cause seizures and, in large amounts, death. Cooked ginkgo seeds are eaten in Asia. The seeds do not contain ginkgolides and flavonoids; they do not have therapeutic effects.

Claims

There is a very diffuse and popular literature, but the hard evidence with PS supplements is limited. Some good evidence supports the efficacy of GB in peripheral vascular disease in patients with claudication. Supplementation with ginkgo increases the walking distance in most claudicants with peripheral vascular diseases. However, standards, management protocols and dosages are not clear and need a full evaluation.

Ginkgo has been used in people with dementia. Benefits in dementia are really difficult to show: in a recent clinical trial, ginkgo was not effective in reducing the progression of dementia and Alzheimer's disease in older people. But then, nothing is really effective in these conditions. It is a wrong, impossible model to test a supplement. Previous US trial indicated that ginkgo supplementation temporarily stabilized mental and social functions in people with mild to moderate dementia. These indications are controversial and effects may be very marginal. But for many people, there is no real drug alternative or treatments.

Other studies show that supplementation with ginkgo does not seem alleviate memory loss (nothing can do it), tinnitus or altitude sickness. Ginkgo may prevent some damage to the kidneys caused by the immunosuppressant cyclosporine. Retinal arterial flow can be improved with supplementation. Also, the microcirculation appears to be affected by ginkgo supplements, but the clinical efficacy of these microcirculatory effects is not available. Ginkgo powder (from dried leaves) appears to improve the healing of vascular ulcerations (venous and diabetics).

Adverse effects

Nausea, dyspepsia, headache, dizziness, heart palpitations may occur with high dosages in some individuals. Ginkgo may theoretically interact with aspirin, NSAIDs, antiplatelet agents and anticoagulants (but there is no definite evidence) and may reduce the efficacy of some anticonvulsants. Ginkgo inhibits monoamine oxidase; patients using some antidepressants (such as monoamine oxidase inhibitors (MAOIs) and selective serotonin reuptake inhibitors (SSRIs)) may have side effects including an increased risk of developing serotonin syndrome, a life-threatening condition.

Ginseng

Ginseng is a family of plants. The term "ginseng" defines any one of 11 species of slow-growing perennial plants with fleshy roots, belonging

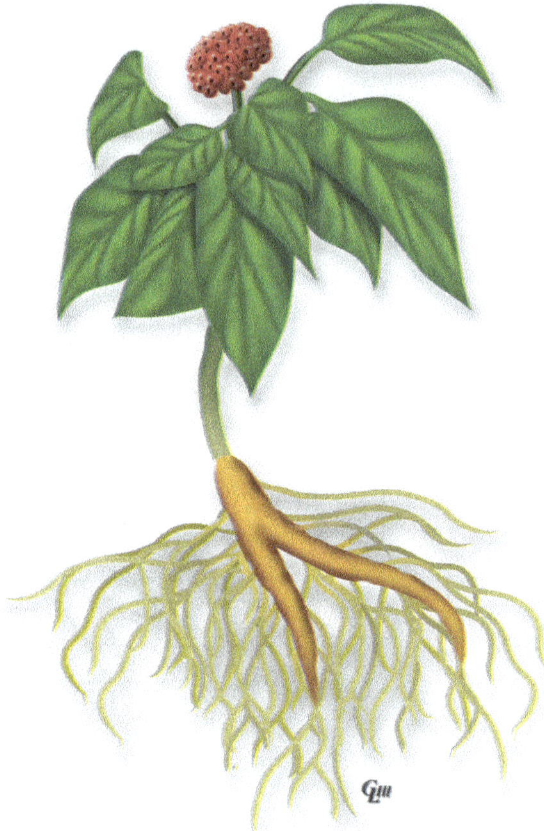

Figure 14: Ginseng.

to the genus *Panax* of the family *Araliaceae*. Supplements are derived from American ginseng (*Panax quinquefolius*) or Asian ginseng. Siberian ginseng is a different genus and does not contain the ingredients believed to be active in the two forms used in supplements (Figure 14).

Ginseng can be used as a fresh product or as dried roots, extracts, solutions, capsules, tablets, sodas, and teas or used in cosmetics. PS supplements are available. Active ingredients in American ginseng are panaxosides (saponin glycosides). Active ingredients in Asian ginseng are ginsenosides (triterpenoid glycosides). Ginseng products vary considerably in quality because many contain little or no detectable active ingredient. In a few cases, some ginseng products from Asia have been purposefully mixed with mandrake root, which has been used to induce vomiting, or with the drugs phenylbutazone or aminopyrazine. These drugs have been removed from the US market because of significant adverse effects.

Claims

Ginsenosides, unique compounds of the *Panax* species, are under basic and clinical research. Siberian ginseng used daily may increase the number of white blood cells and the activity of the T cells as well as the cytotoxic T cells and natural killer cells that eliminate invading cells and those that have been virally infected.

A study has shown that in patients with herpes simplex virus 2 (which can lead to genital herpes), there was a reduction (of 50%) in the number of outbreaks. The outbreaks that occurred were less severe and did not last as long. Ginseng contains significant levels of phytoestrogens. This problem has not been evaluated as much as is required; it needs further investigation.

Red ginseng (*hóng shēn*), *P. ginseng*, is peeled, heated through steaming at standard boiling temperatures of 100°C (212°F) and then dried or sun-dried. It is frequently marinated in an herbal brew which results in the root becoming extremely brittle. Ginseng extracts and supplements are commonly used according to legendary popular, historical beliefs to enhance physical (including sexual) and mental performance; ginseng is said to have adaptogenic effects (i.e., it may increase energy and resistance to the harmful effects of stress and aging).

Other claims include reduction of plasma glucose levels, increases in high-density lipoprotein (HDL), hemoglobin and protein levels. The report of a stimulation of the immune system with a possible anticancer effect borders science fiction. Cardiotonic, endocrine, CNS and estrogenic effects are possibly weak and of an extremely limited clinical value. Studies have shown that Asian ginseng lowers glucose with possible beneficial effects on immunity. There is no evidence for other health claims. A recent study indicates that a polysaccharide extract of *P. quinquefolius* may be useful in helping prevent colds.

Adverse effects

Anxiety, nervousness and excitability may occur (on an individual basis); these effects decrease after a few days of use. Improvement in concentration may decrease, plasma glucose may become lower (causing hypoglycemia). Ginseng has a significant estrogen-like effect; therefore, pregnant women or women who are breastfeeding should not use it; it should also be avoided in children. Rare reports include other side effects (such as asthma attacks, increased blood pressure, palpitations, and in postmenopausal women, uterine bleeding).

For many people, ginseng taste is unpleasant. Ginseng supplements (considering the dosage) can interact with antihyperglycemic drugs, aspirin, NSAIDs, corticosteroids, digoxin, estrogens, MAOIs, and anticoagulants. A characteristic symptom of acute overdose of *P. ginseng* is bleeding. Symptoms of milder overdose may include dry mouth and lips, excitation, fidgeting, irritability, tremor, palpitations, blurred vision, headache, insomnia, increased body temperature, increased blood pressure, edema, decreased appetite, dizziness, itching, eczema, early morning diarrhea, bleeding and fatigue.

Gross overdose with *P. ginseng* may include nausea, vomiting, irritability, restlessness, urinary and bowel incontinence, fever, increased blood pressure, increased respiration, decreased sensitivity and reaction to light, decreased heart rate, cyanotic (blue) facial complexion, red facial complexion, seizures, convulsions and delirium.

Glucosamine

In the US, glucosamine is one of the most common nonvitamin, nonmineral supplements used by adults. It is a very well-studied and known supplement with several PS supplements available. Glucosamine ($C_6H_{13}NO_5$) is an amino sugar and a precursor in the biochemical synthesis of glycosylated proteins and lipids.

Glucosamine is part of the structure of the polysaccharides chitosan and chitin, the main structural components of exoskeletons of crustaceans and other arthropods (also found in the cell walls of fungi and many higher organisms). Glucosamine is a precursor or multiple-cartilage constituent. It is extracted from chitin (from shells of crabs, oysters and shrimp) and is used in tablet or capsule form, usually as glucosamine sulfate but sometimes as glucosamine hydrochloride. Glucosamine supplements often include chondroitin sulfate.

Claims

Glucosamine as for other, heavily marketed supplements claims part of the possible benefits on laboratory studies that are of difficult interpretation and clinical meaning. Some clinical studies are controversial with some trials reporting symptomatic relief from arthritic pain and good effects on stiffness; some larger studies report minimal benefit in comparison with placebo. The effects should be considered on the basis of clinical conditions, presence of inflammation, age, dosages and so many other factors that cannot allow a generalization.

There is no evidence to date that supplementation with glucosamine in athletes and sport participants may prevent or limit joint damage or improve recovery after an injury. According to the *Merck Manual*, a strong evidence supports the use of glucosamine sulfate PS supplements in the management and treatment of mild–moderate symptomatic OA of the knee (usually associated to degeneration and partly to inflammation). Short-term effects tend to affect signs/symptoms and have a role in the treatment of severe knee OA.

A longer supplementation (possibly >6 months) may positively alter the evolution of osteoarthritis even modulating the regrowth of cartilage. The effects of glucosamine on OA in other anatomical locations (i.e., fingers) or in arthritis and in conditions with a strong inflammatory component (and in younger subjects) are less defined. Some evidence suggests glucosamine has both analgesic and anti-inflammatory disease-modifying effects. However, evidence from large and studies still shows limited and individualized benefit.

One large study indicated that glucosamine hydrochloride is more beneficial when combined with chondroitin sulfate. The mechanisms are unknown; improvements may be related to improved glycosaminoglycan synthesis due to the sulfate components. The usual recommended dose is 500 mg per os tid. With supplementation, glucosamine concentrations in plasma and synovial fluid increase significantly from baseline levels and the levels in the two fluids are generally highly correlated. These levels could be biologically advantageous to articular cartilage. However, the levels are still 10–100 fold lower than what is theoretically required to improve the cartilage (chondrocytes) and to build new tissue. Glucosamine sulfate uptake in synovial fluid may be as much as 20%, or could be negligible, indicating minimal biological or clinical significance.

Adverse effects

Allergy has been observed (i.e., in patients who have shellfish allergy); dyspepsia, fatigue, insomnia, headache, some photosensitivity and occasional nail changes may occur. Concerns about the use in diabetics have been suggested. However, the effects of oral administration of large doses of glucosamine in animals, and the effects of glucosamine supplementation with normal recommended dosages in humans, indicate that glucosamine does not cause glucose intolerance and has no documented effects on glucose metabolism.

Other studies conducted in lean or obese subjects concluded that oral glucosamine at standard doses does not cause or significantly worsen insulin resistance or endothelial dysfunction. There have been few interactions between glucosamine and other medications; the most significant interaction has been reported with anticoagulants. FDA and WHO medication programs have reported multiple cases with elevated (above safety levels) international normalized ratio (INR) in individuals using anticoagulants. Caution should be used when anticoagulants and glucosamine are used.

In the US, glucosamine is not approved by the FDA for medical use. Glucosamine is classified as a supplement; therefore, standards, safety and formulation are the exclusive responsibility of the manufacturer. Evidence of safety or efficacy is not required as long as it is not advertised or "claimed" as a treatment for a defined medical condition. The NIH is evaluating supplementation with glucosamine in obese patients, since this population may be particularly sensitive to any possible effects of glucosamine on insulin resistance.

In most of Europe, glucosamine is approved as a drug and sold in the form of glucosamine sulfate. Evidence of safety and efficacy is required for the medical use of glucosamine as for any other drug, and guidelines have recommended its use as an effective and safe therapy for OA.

Goldenseal

Goldenseal, an endangered US plant, is related to the buttercup. Its active components are hydrastine and berberine, which have antiseptic activity. Berberine also has shown antidiarrheal properties (Figure 15).

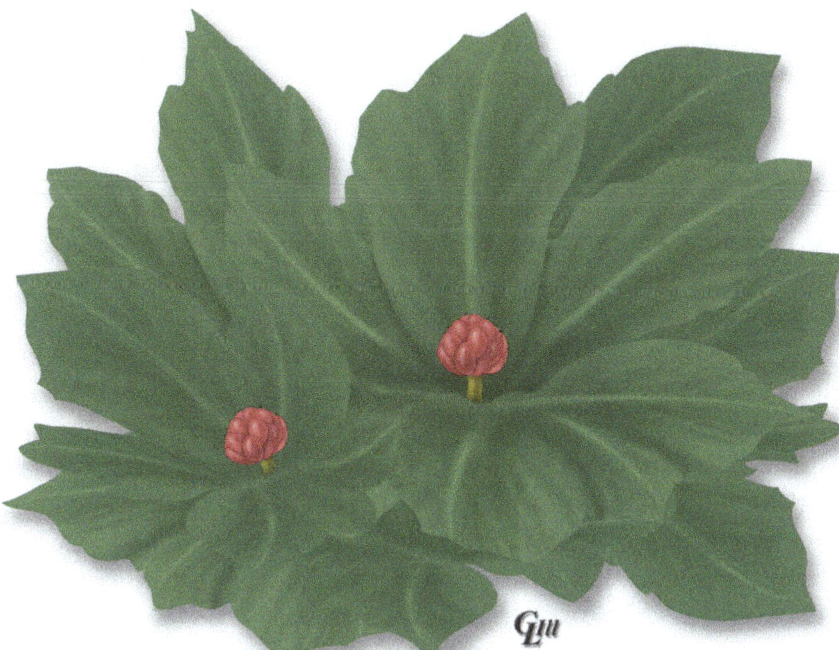

Figure 15: Goldenseal.

Claims

Goldenseal is used as an antiseptic wash for mouth sores, inflamed and sore eyes, irritated skin and as a douche for vaginal infections. It has been combined with *Echinacea* as a cold remedy, but the efficacy of goldenseal as a cold remedy has not been proved. Goldenseal is also used as a remedy for indigestion and diarrhea. In two relatively well-designed studies, berberine isolated from goldenseal has been seen to reduce diarrhea.

Adverse effects

Goldenseal may have many adverse effects, including nausea, anxiety, dyspepsia, uterine contractions, jaundice in neonates and worsening of hypertension. If used in large amounts, goldenseal can cause seizures and respiratory failure and may even affect contraction of the heart. Goldenseal may — theoretically — interact with warfarin. Women who are pregnant or breastfeeding, neonates and people who have seizure disorders or problems with blood clotting should not be treated with goldenseal. Berberine may reduce the anticoagulant effect of heparin.

Grape leaf

Vitis vinifera (common grape vine) is a species of *Vitis*, native to the Mediterranean region, central Europe, and southwestern Asia. Grape leaves may boost the intake of vitamins being a rich source of the fat-soluble vitamins A and K. A one-cup serving of grape leaves contains 3,853 international units of vitamin A (corresponding to 1 d of recommended intake). A cup of grape leaves also contains 15.2 μg of vitamin K, 17% of the recommended intake for women or 13% for men. Grape leaves also provide calcium and iron.

Medical applications of grape leaf extracts and PS supplements are limited. Grape leaves are mildly anti-inflammatory compounds. Chronic inflammation is associated to several conditions (heart disease, many types of cancer, Alzheimer's disease). Other diseases that are associated to inflammation include arthritis and many GI diseases, such as Crohn's disease. Grape leaves are full of nutrients and have a low glycemic index. According to a study conducted (by the Dermatology at the University of

Freiburg), a grape leaf PS supplement may control edema and some symptoms in patients with CVI.

Other uses

Grape leaves — particularly red grape leaves — have been used in the treatment of diarrhea, menstrual bleeding, uterine hemorrhage, some sores and excess vaginal discharge. Native Americans made grape leaves into a tea for diarrhea, hepatitis, stomachaches and pains. Grape leaves have a history of being used for a wide variety of conditions, but more research is needed to determine their true efficacy.

Grape seed

Grape seed extracts and PS supplements derivate from whole grape seeds that have a great concentration of vitamin E, flavonoids, linoleic acid and phenolic procyanidins (known as OPCs or oligomeric procyanidins). The typical commercial opportunity of extracting grape seed constituents has been for chemicals known as polyphenols having antioxidant activity. An important polyphenol contained in grape seeds is resveratrol, which is under evaluation (actually it has been for years) for its possible cardiovascular, antiaging and anticancer effects.

Other preliminary research on disease models include management of skin ulcers and wounds as OPCs induce the production of vascular endothelial growth factor and accelerated healing. In bone physiology, grape seed extracts and PS supplements appear to enhance density and strength (but most work is in animal studies). OPCs may have antiviral and antibacterial activity. A recent study has shown efficacy of a grape seed PS supplement in normalizing in a short period of time blood pressure in borderline hypertensives.

One study in patients with coronary disease and cardiac risk factors found that 4 weeks of grape seed supplementation caused a minimal improvement in endothelial function (for what it may mean from a clinical point of view). A meta-analysis of grape seed supplementation confirms that grape seed significantly lowers systolic blood pressure and decreases heart rate with minimal effects on lipids. The study included different patients with different supplements and has a limited clinical meaning.

Adverse effects

Grape seed PS supplements are used in capsules or tablets usually containing 50 or 100 mg. Because of the possible action of proanthocyanidins on decreasing platelet adhesion (in theory), grape seed supplement may theoretically act on coagulation, increasing clotting time. Grape seed supplements are also an aromatase inhibitor and may suppress the conversion of testosterone to estradiol, but this effect may require high loads.

Green tea

Green tea is made from the leaves from *Camellia sinensis* that have undergone minimal oxidation during processing. Green tea originated in China, but it has become associated with many cultures throughout Asia. Green tea is made from the dried leaves of the same plant as traditional tea, an evergreen shrub (Figure 16).

Traditional tea leaves are fermented, and green tea leaves are steamed but unfermented. Green tea may be brewed and drunk or ingested in extracted tablet or capsule form in PS supplements. It has multiple components that are thought to have antioxidant and, theoretically, anticancer effects. Green tea contains polyphenols and catechins as well as caffeine, but many extracts have been decaffeinated. Green tea contains a variety of enzymes, amino acids, carbohydrates, lipids, sterols, related compounds, phytochemicals, and dietary minerals.

The many claims that have been made for the health benefits of green tea are based on its chemical composition and defined both in *in vitro* and *in vivo* human studies. Consuming large volumes of green tea, and particularly of green tea extracts, may lead to oxidative stress and liver toxicity. There is no good evidence that green tea helps to prevent or treat cancer. A recent study has indicated that a PS supplement helps to effectively control the metabolic syndrome in a group of otherwise healthy subjects in a few weeks.

Claims

Green tea is said to have multiple health benefits, none of which are supported by strong scientific evidence. It has been used for cancer prevention, weight loss, serum lipid reduction, prevention of coronary

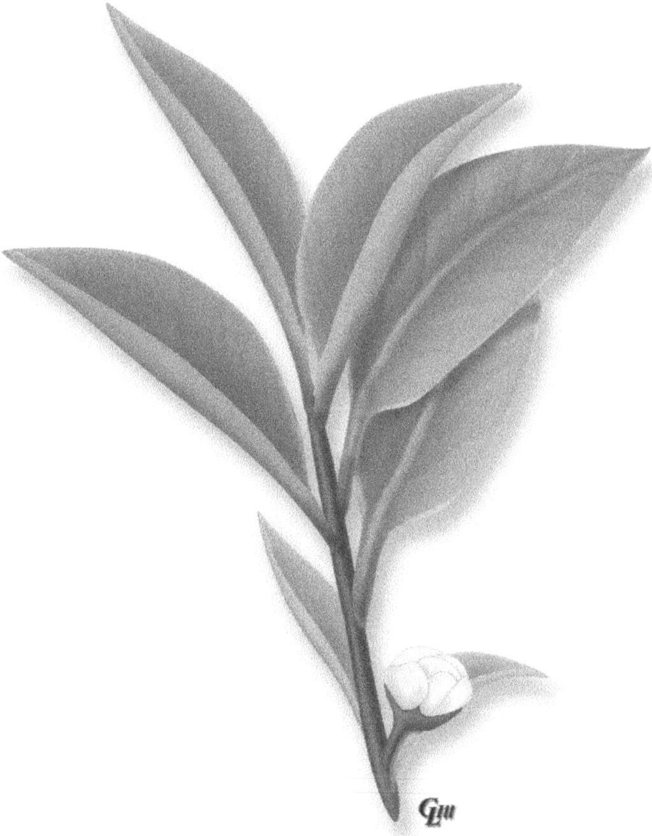

Figure 16: Green tea.

artery disease, memory enhancement, relief of OA, pain, treatment of menopausal symptoms and longevity.

Adverse effects

Adverse effects are mostly related to the similar effects of caffeine. They include insomnia, anxiety, tachycardia and mild tremor. Pregnant women should avoid excessive caffeine. Green tea may interfere with the anticancer drug bortezomib (Velcade®) and other boronic-acid-based proteasome inhibitors.

Licorice

Licorice is the root of *Glycyrrhiza glabra*. A sweet flavor can be extracted from the root. The licorice plant is a legume that is native to southern Europe, India and parts of Asia. It is not botanically related to anise, star anise, or fennel, which include similar flavoring compounds. Natural licorice has a very characteristic and sweet taste has been used medicinally as capsules, tablets or extracts (Figure 17). Most licorice candies are flavored artificially and do not contain natural licorice. Glycyrrhizin is the active

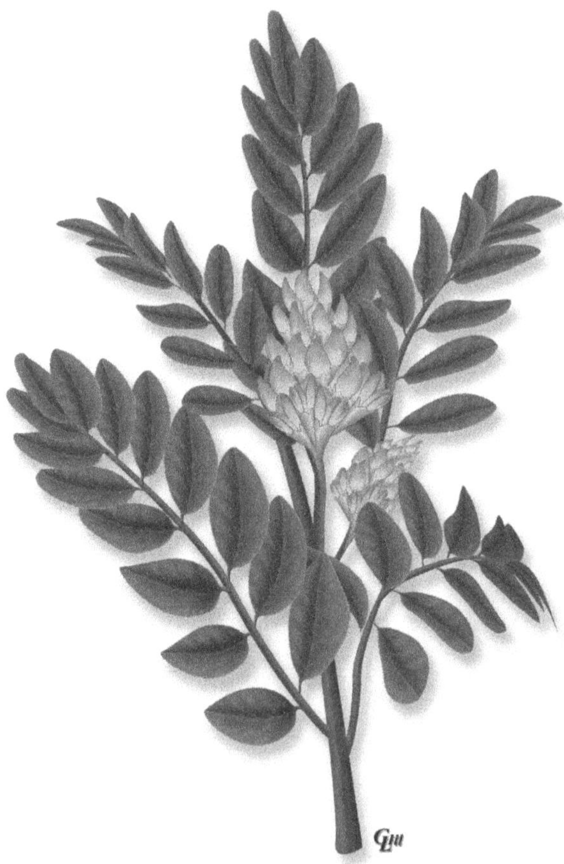

Figure 17: Licorice.

ingredient in natural licorice. For people sensitive to the effects of glycyrrhizin, products that contain a much lower amount of glycyrrhizin (about one tenth) are available (deglycyrrhizinated licorice).

Claims

Licorice may help to control or suppress coughs, to sooth a sore throat and to relieve stomach upset. When applied topically, it is said to improve skin irritation and eczema. There are not enough studies to define whether licorice is effective for improving stomach ulcers of complications associated to hepatitis C. This supplement has been proposed as being useful for liver protection in tuberculosis therapy, but there is no evidence. Licorice may be effective in controlling hyperlipidemia, and some studies showed some efficacy in treating inflammation-induced skin hyperpigmentation.

Licorice may also be effective in preventing some neurodegenerative disorders and even dental caries. The laxative, antidiabetic, anti-inflammatory, immunomodulatory and antitumoral activities are under evaluation: the expectorant properties of licorice have also been under investigation with conflicting results. Licorice is popular in Italy (particularly in the South) and Spain in its natural form. The root of the plant is simply dug up, washed and chewed. Throughout Italy, unsweetened licorice is consumed in the form of small black pieces made only from 100% pure licorice extract; the taste is bitter and intense. In these forms, it is not a supplement but just a candy.

Adverse effects

High doses of licorice (>1 oz a day) and glycyrrhizin may cause renal Na and water retention even leading to higher blood pressure and potassium excretion. This may cause low potassium levels. Increased potassium excretion may become a problem for patients with heart disease if they use digoxin or diuretics that increase potassium excretion. These patients should avoid licorice. Licorice may increase the risk of premature delivery; pregnant women should avoid licorice. The isoflavene glabrene and the isoflavane glabridin, found in the roots of licorice, are phytoestrogens.

Melatonin

Melatonin, the jet-setter status symbol, is also a hormone produced by the pineal gland. It helps in regulating circadian rhythm and sleep. It is derived from animal sources, but it can also be produced synthetically.

In some countries, melatonin is considered a drug and is regulated as such; *5-methoxytryptamine* is a hormone found in animals, plants, fungi and bacteria. It is the most fundamental and universal hormone in the evolution of cellular life, primarily acting as an antioxidant against the Sun's radiation. It is synthesized in animal cells directly from the amino acid tryptophan, but in other organisms through the Shikimic acid pathway, in response to dark–light periods (photoperiod).

Melatonin is categorized by the FDA as a supplement. It is sold over the counter in the US and Canada without any regulation as a pharmaceutical drug. FDA regulations applying to medications are not applicable to melatonin. However, FDA rules required that by June 2010, all production of dietary supplements must comply with "current Good Manufacturing Practices" (cGMP) and be manufactured with "controls that result in a consistent product free of contamination, with accurate labelling". The industry has also been required to report to the FDA all serious adverse events, and the FDA has (within the cGMP guidelines) begun enforcement of that requirement.

Claims

Some (weak) scientific evidence suggests the use of melatonin to minimize the effects of jet lag, especially in people travelling eastward over two to five time zones. In one large study, melatonin supplements did not relieve symptoms of jet lag; at the moment, only a few small studies suggest that these supplements can treat insomnia. Melatonin can be taken orally as capsules, tablets or liquid. It is also available in a form to be used sublingually, and there are transdermal patches.

Standard dosage is not established and ranges from 0.5 to 5 mg po taken 1 h before usual bedtime on the day of travel and two to four nights after arrival. The evidence supporting use of melatonin as a sleep aid in adults and children with neuropsychiatric disorders (e.g., pervasive developmental disorders) is weak. Melatonin has also been studied as a potential treatment of gastroesophageal reflux, some immune disorders, depression, seasonal affective disorder (SAD), circadian rhythm sleep disorders and even sexual dysfunction and insomnia in the elderly with limited results.

Melatonin can alter electrophysiological processes associated with memory, such as long-term potentiation (LTP). Melatonin has been tested in Alzheimer's disease. Supplementation with melatonin is considered a possible and effective preventive treatment for migraines and cluster headaches.

Adverse effects

Hangover, drowsiness, headache and transient depression are adverse effects that may occur in some subjects. Melatonin may worsen depression. Theoretically, prion infection caused by products derived from neurologic tissues of animals is a risk. Melatonin can lower follicle-stimulating hormone (FSH) levels. Effects of the hormone on human reproduction remain unclear, although it was with some effect tried as a contraceptive in the 1990s. Symptoms of Parkinson's disease may be affected.

Milk thistle

Milk thistle (MT) is a purple-flowered plant. *Silybum marianum* has other common names including *Carduus marianus*, MT, blessed MT, Marian thistle, Mary thistle, Saint Mary's thistle, Mediterranean MT, variegated thistle and Scotch thistle. This species is an annual or biennial plant of the Asteraceae family. Its sap and seeds contain the active ingredient silymarin, a potent antioxidant and hepatotropic agent. The extracts include some 65–80% silymarin (a flavonolignan complex) and 20–35% fatty acids, including linoleic acid (Figure 18).

Silymarin is a complex mixture of polyphenolic molecules, including seven closely related flavonolignans (silybin A, silybin B, isosilybin A, isosilybin B, silychristin, isosilychristin, silydianin) and one major flavonoid (taxifolin). Silibinin, a semipurified fraction of silymarin, is primarily a mixture of two diastereoisomers, silybin A and silybin B, in an approximately 1:1 ratio. Silibinin (silymarin I) appears to have many significant hepatoprotective, hepatotropic activities. and antihepatotoxic

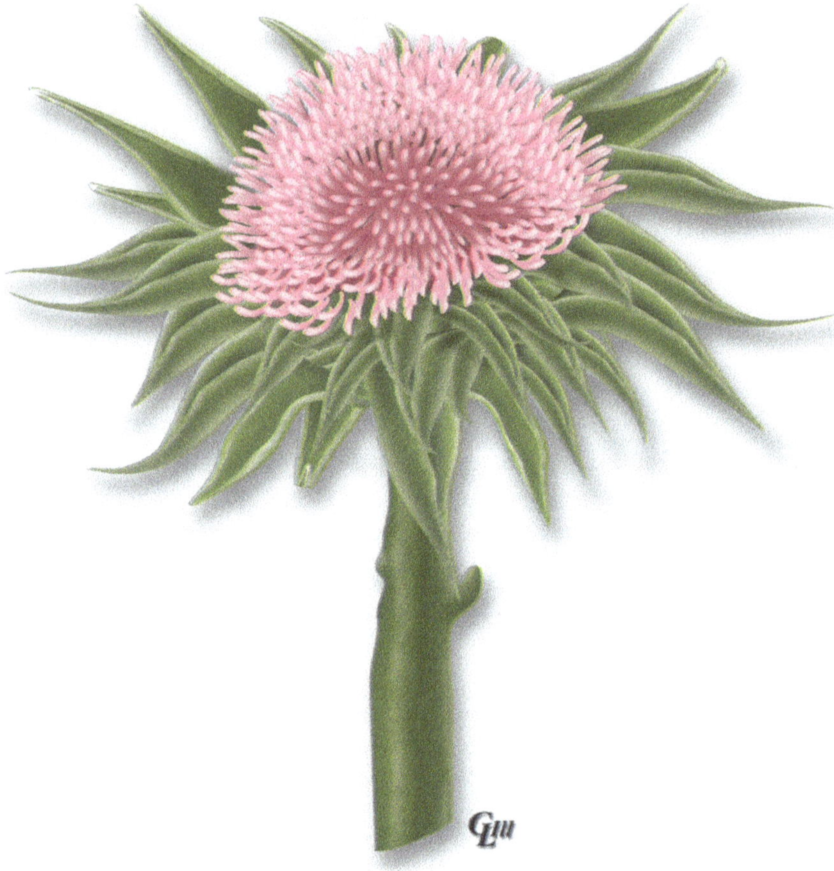

Figure 18: Milk thistle.

activities that may protect liver cells against some toxins. *In vitro* research has indicated that that silibinin is hepatoprotective.

MT extracts and PS supplements both prevent and repair damage to the liver from toluene and/or xylene. Workers exposed to toxic vapors from toluene or xylene for years used a PS MT supplement with 80% silymarin for 30 d. The workers using the supplement showed significant improvement in liver function tests (ALT and AST) and platelet counts. A study in 2010 found that eight major compounds in silybum, including seven flavonolignans — silybin A, silybin B, isosilybin A, isosilybin B, silychristin, isosilychristin, silydianin — and one flavonoid, taxifolin, are inhibitors of HCV RNA-dependent RNA polymerase, suggesting a significant potential in specifically treating liver damage linked to hepatitis C. Silymarin supplementation (140 mg os tid) appears to have limited effects when used for 1 y in combination with ursodeoxycholic acid (UDCA) in the management of primary biliary cirrhosis.

MT supplementation was associated with a trend toward reducing some liver-damaging effects of chemotherapy in a study involving 50 children. In clinical studies, silymarin has typically been used in oral doses ranging from 420 to 480 mg/d (in two to three divided doses). Higher doses have been evaluated (600 mg daily in the treatment of patients with type 2 diabetes and 600–1,200 mg daily in patients with chronic hepatitis C). Optimization of dosage, solubility and administration plans have not been defined. MT (with dandelion and other extracts) has been considered a hangover cure as the bitter tincture may help organs to eliminate it after heavy drinking.

Claims

MT is said to treat cirrhosis (or control its evolution) and to protect the liver from viral hepatitis. Also, it may attenuate the damaging effects of alcohol and protect liver from the effects of some hepatotoxic drugs. In *in vitro* studies, silymarin increases the levels of intrahepatic glutathione, an antioxidant considered important for detoxification. Studies have been unable to show that MT PS supplements offer significant benefits to people with liver disease. However, the studies should focus on very specific conditions as the causes of liver damage can be really too many, and very often there is more than one cause.

There are individual case reports that claim fatality reduction in acute mushroom poisoning. Results indicate that severe liver damage due to *Amanita phalloides* liver cell necrosis can be prevented effectively when administration of silybin begins within 48 h of mushroom intake. Other case control studies also suggest that silibinin reduces mortality from mushroom poisoning. Other uses to be clinically verified indicate that MT supplementation may lower cholesterol levels, reduce cell damage caused by radiation (and chemotherapy), reduce insulin resistance in people with type 2 diabetes with cirrhosis, reduce the growth of some cancer cells (breast, cervical, prostate cancers) and even have some effects in patients with Alzheimer's disease (both in prevention and treatment). However, studies and results are very limited.

A recent Indian multicenter study on more than 650 patients in different levels and conditions associated with liver damage indicated that a new PS supplement (liverubin) is generally effective in decreasing liver damage (considering enzymes) in weeks without any side effect. Another study in moderate, temporary liver damage also has shown the efficacy of the same supplement. A potential positive action of PS supplements could be considered when giving patients drugs or treatments that may potentially cause liver damage or when patients are at higher risk of liver damage.

Adverse effects

No significant adverse effects have been reported with MT PS supplements. MT may increase the effects of antihyperglycemic drugs and may theoretically interfere with indinavir. Women with hormone-sensitive conditions (breast, uterine and ovarian cancer, endometriosis and uterine fibroids) should avoid MT supplements.

NKCP® (nattokinase)

NKCP® (nattokinase) is a purified filtrate of *Bacillus subtilis* natto culture. Natto is a traditional Japanese food made with *fermented soybeans*. The *Bacillus subtilis* natto (formed in the fermentation process) produce a functional proteins (including nattokinase) which maintain optimum blood viscosity and thrombogenicity. Nattokinase helps reduce the risk of thrombosis possibly in both the arterial and venous circulation. Deep vein thrombosis (DVT) occurring during or after long flights may be partially prevented by nattokinase.

Natto as a food may contain large amounts of vitamin K_2 which may interfere with warfarin. NKCP® (nattokinase, Daiwa) is a specific PS supplement of natto *Bacillus* culture (Bacillopeptidase F) used (tablets 125 mg) for preventing thrombosis. Several enzymes have been identified in NKCP®, including nattokinase. These enzymes inactivate in the blood plasminogen activator inhibitor (PAI-1) which tends to increase with age. By reducing PAI-1, NKCP® increases the efficiency of blood control mechanisms associated with viscosity. NKCP® does not directly act upon blood viscosity and does not dissolve blood clots. The supplement increases the efficiency of blood-control mechanisms including spontaneous fibrinolysis. Therefore, NKCP® does not alter normal blood coagulation or platelet aggregation.

Safety: NKCP® nattokinase safety has been evaluated in clinical studies. No clinical adverse effects were seen with dosages between 750 and 1,250 mg/d. A dose of 250–500 mg of NKCP® (2–4 tablets) is recommended as the standard dose per day (after the evening meal).

NKCP® has a thrombolytic effect *in vitro* and *in vivo* after ingestion. The effect is milder when compared to the plasminogen activator (t-PA). NKCP® has been confirmed to decompose and inactivate plasminogen activator inhibitor (PAI-1) in cell culture systems.

Oral NKCP® administration reduces the plasminogen activator inhibitor (PAI-1) and helps the plasminogen activator (t-PA) to work more efficiently; t-PA activates plasmin and reduces blood fibrin. Therefore, NKCP® facilitates the activation of the spontaneous fibrinolysis cascade by reducing PAI-1 and maintains the balance between coagulation and fibrinolysis. NKCP® ingestion is unlikely to dissolve fibrin excessively causing clinical problems (i.e., bleeding). NKCP® ingestion is unlikely to cause unexpected fibrinolysis.

Nattokinase NKCP® has been used to prevent thrombosis in long flights (in association with Pycnogenol® (see the next section) in a specific combination defined as "Flite Tabs®"). NKCP® has also been used to prevent recurrent DVT after an episode of major DVT and for the prevention of new episodes of retinal thrombosis. However, data (on file) are not widely available.

Pycnogenol®

In his Berlin laboratories, Charles Haimoff developed a unique substance, a water-soluble flavonoid extract from the bark of the French maritime pine tree, called Pycnogenol®. Pycnogenol® extract (unique, PS standardized supplement) is a potent blend of antioxidants, a natural anti-inflammatory agent. It stimulates the generation of collagen and hyaluronic acid and improves the natural vasomotor activity of blood vessels by supporting production of nitric oxide. It is one of the most studied supplements and it is considered a case model for all PS supplements development and evaluation (Figure 19).

(a)

(b)

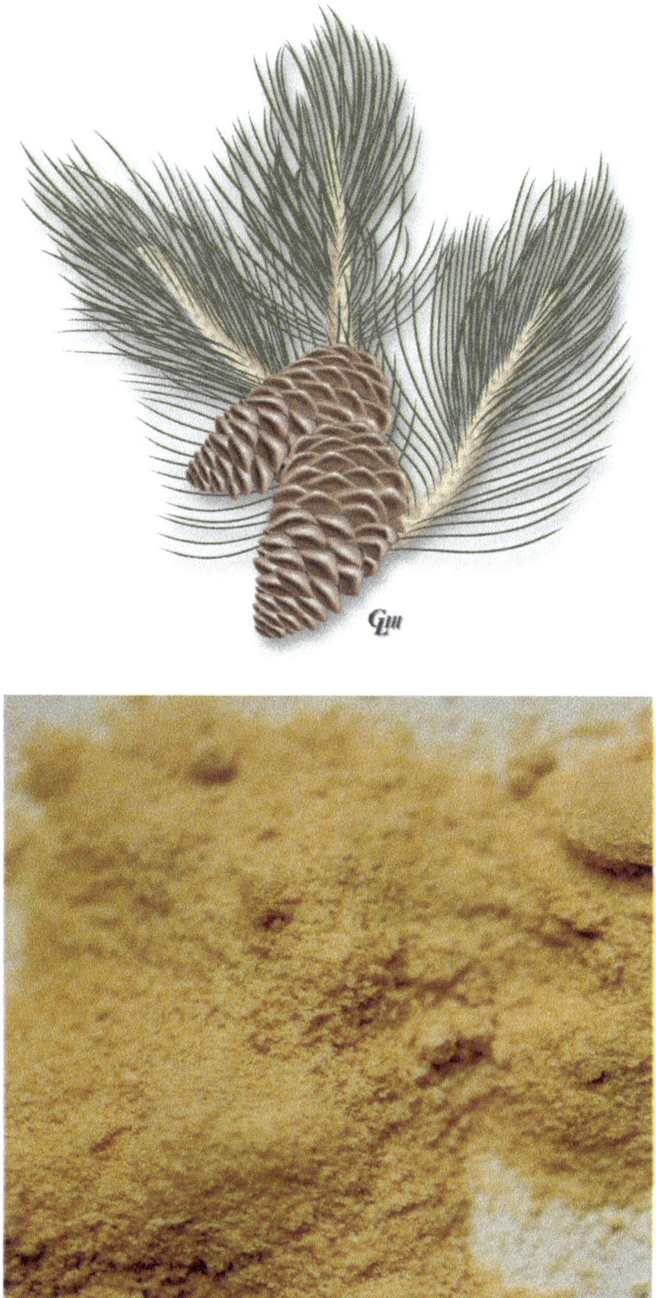

Figure 19: Pycnogenol® (a) plant and (b) powder.

Pycnogenol® helps in maintaining a physiological circulation by improving the relaxation of arteries according to physiological needs. Consequently, Pycnogenol® improves perfusion in many organs and modulates blood pressure. The antioxidant activity of Pycnogenol® protects the skin from the free radicals produced by UV exposure and environmental damage. Pycnogenol® has been tested in arthrosis; it improves joint mobility and flexibility, and its anti-inflammatory activity helps in relieving signs/symptoms associated to both degenerative and inflammatory arthrosis.

Pycnogenol® has been used to improve retinal circulation — reducing edema — in diabetics with microangiopathy. Supplementation with Pycnogenol® controls some cardiovascular risk factors with improvement in blood pressure in borderline hypertensive subjects and modulates platelet adhesion. Also blood lipids and blood sugar values may be improved in most cardiovascular subjects with a positive interaction with "standard" treatments. Several studies show the effects of Pycnogenol® supplementation in controlling most cardiovascular risk factors. Circulation studies have found that this supplement increases the induced vasodilation of arteries (when altered) in cardiovascular patients.

Blood pressure studies in hypertensives have shown that Pycnogenol® improves the physiological vasodilatory response after reactive hyperemia. It has a positive interaction with any other drug used to control risk factors. With Pycnogenol®, cholesterol may be reduced in selected cardiovascular patients and in most subjects at risk. Supplementation with Pycnogenol® tends to increase HDL cholesterol.

The supplement has also shown an important activity in subjects with arthrosis by improving symptoms in association with lowering inflammatory markers and oxidative stress. In these patients, Pycnogenol® limits the activation of the proinflammatory NF-κB. As a consequence, subjects treated with this PS supplement generate less matrix metalloproteinase (MMP) enzymes (responsible for the degeneration of cartilage collagen in OA). The supplement also inhibits the generation of COX-2 enzymes in inflammation, lowering pain.

In sports, Pycnogenol® has shown efficacy in improving physical performance; athletes showed an increase of endurance with the supplement. In one study, the athletes performed under controlled conditions (on a treadmill). The study showed a significant increase of endurance with Pycnogenol®. The supplement also improves muscle recovery and muscular pain associated to fatigue and alleviates the occurrence of cramps. In venous disease (uncomplicated VV) and in CVI, Pycnogenol® improves edema — the hallmark of CVI — that may progress to more serious complications (including ulceration) if left untreated.

At least 15 clinical studies have been published on venous insufficiency and CVI. In this field, Pycnogenol® has a very strong documentation. The higher efficacy of Pycnogenol® as a venous insufficiency management and treatment tool (in comparison with other products) is obvious in several studies. Pycnogenol® is more effective than horse chestnut extracts, but it is also comparatively more effective than any other treatment for CVI with a power factor of 10 (a dose some 10 times higher is needed for other products to have some effects, comparable to the effects produced by Pycnogenol®). It produces more significant results on CVI symptoms than any other product.

This supplement also reduces edema due to long flights. Long periods of immobility, dry environment, small airplane cabin space are contributing factors to leg swelling due to limited venous circulation; fluids tend to accumulate in distal tissues. Leg and ankle swelling are also associated to vein thrombosis.

Recent studies on flight-related swelling found that Pycnogenol® has a positive effect on leg swelling and edema during long flights lasting 7–12 h. More recent studies on cognitive functions and an acute model study on jet lag, associated to some cognitive impairment, indicate an improvement in cognitive functions in healthy individuals. This observation may be physiologically related to the control of water (and edema) within the cerebral tissue. Tinnitus and Meniere's syndrome have been improved in more limited studies by supplementation with Pycnogenol®.

Two other studies have indicated that Pycnogenol® supplementation may reduce the course of common cold of at least 1 d and reduce the incidence of tracheal and pulmonary complications. Also studies on asthma and psoriasis have shown very interesting results. The product behaves as a general, natural anti-inflammatory agent and effectively controls the genesis and evolution of edema (including subclinical edema) associated to several clinical conditions. Several applications with different dosages (30–200 ng/d) have been made available. Microcirculation has also been selectively evaluated in several studies that have indicated its efficacy (i.e., in diabetic microangiopathy and vasospastic conditions).

Recent studies have indicated that Pycnogenol® may slow down the progression of atherosclerotic plaques in selected individuals and the progression from asymptomatic to symptomatic cardiovascular stages in subjects with more significant, stenotic plaques. The atherosclerosis study is still in progress, and it is very promising. This study uses a combination of Pycnogenol® and TTFCA. Pycnogenol® is now available in thin skin patches also. Initial results indicate an important anti-inflammatory action and a decrease in oxidative stress after patch application.

Adverse effects

No clinically significant adverse effect has been observed. The product is very safe and well tolerated, and so far, no significant adverse interactions with other treatments or drugs have been observed.

Quercetin

Quercetin is a flavonol found in many fruits, vegetables, leaves and grains. The name derives from *Quercus*. It is a naturally occurring polar auxin transport inhibitor. Quercetin is present in various kinds of honey from different plant sources. The enzyme quercitrinase can be found in *Aspergillus flavus*. Its substrates are quercitrin and H_2O and releases quercetin and L-rhamnose. It is an enzyme in the rutin catabolic pathway. Quercetin 3-*O*-sulfate is a human plasma quercetin metabolite.

Quercetin is the aglycone form of a number of other flavonoid glycosides, such as rutin and quercitrin, found in citrus fruit, buckwheat and onions. Quercetin forms the glycosides quercitrin and rutin together with rhamnose and rutinose, respectively. CTN-986 is a quercetin derivative found in cottonseeds and cottonseed oil. Miquelianin is the quercetin 3-*O*-β-D-glucuronopyranoside. Quercetin may induce insulin secretion by activation of L-type calcium channels in pancreatic β-cells.

Quercetin is used for empirically treating conditions of the heart including atherosclerosis, high cholesterol and to control cardiovascular risk factors. PS supplements are also used in treatment of subjects with diabetes, cataracts, hay fever, peptic ulcer, schizophrenia, inflammation, asthma, gout, viral infections and in benign prostatic hypertrophy. Quercetin is also used to increase endurance and improve athletic performance with very limited evidence. Quercetin has antioxidant and anti-inflammatory effects that need to be evaluated using PS supplements.

Basically, at the moment, there is no defined clinical or preventive application. The FDA has issued warning letters to emphasize that quercetin is not a defined nutrient, cannot be assigned a dietary content level and is not regulated as a drug to treat any human disease.

Adverse effects

Quercetin is contraindicated with some antibiotics. It may interact with fluoroquinolones (quercetin competitively binds to bacterial DNA gyrase). Whether this inhibits or enhances the effect of fluoroquinolones is not clear. AHFS Drug Information specifically names quercetin as a compound with potential harmful interactions with taxol/paclitaxel. As paclitaxel is metabolized primarily by CYP2C8, its bioavailability may be increased unpredictably, potentially leading to harmful side effects.

Robuvit®

Robuvit® is a new, highly standardized PS supplement produced from a wood extract from French *Quercus robur*. Robuvit® includes several ellagitannins that have significant antioxidant and anti-inflammatory actions with an important effect on distal edema (i.e., in lymphatic patients). Human absorption of specific roburins from a French oak wood extract (Robuvit®) can be measured by evaluating the plasmatic increase of total phenols and the appearance of some roburin metabolites (Figure 20).

(a)

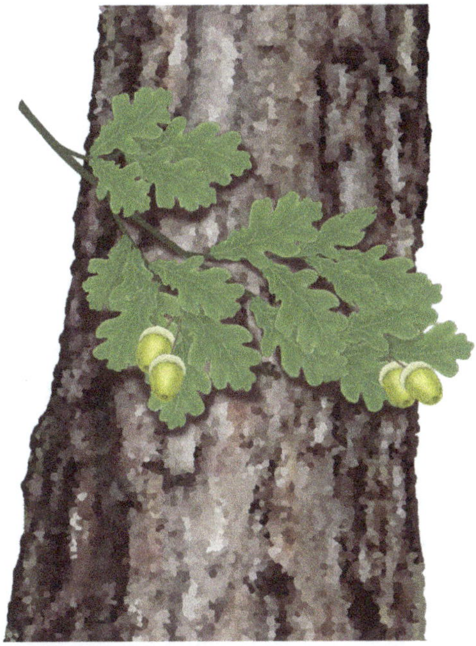

(b)

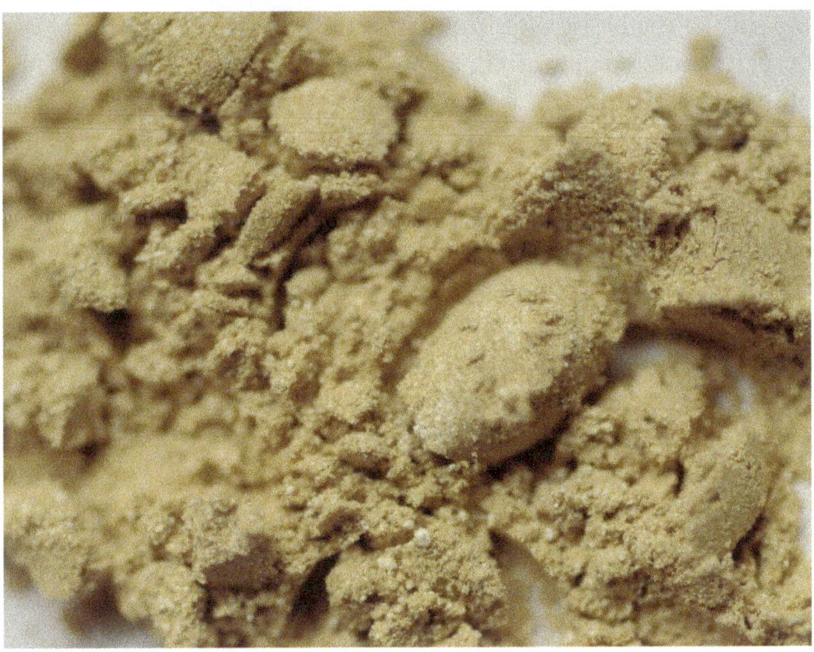

Figure 20: Robuvit® (a) plant and (b) powder.

Supplementation with Robuvit® increases the global plasma antioxidant capacity. Cell cultures have assessed the action of metabolites on gene expression modulation in endothelial, neuronal and keratinocyte cell lines. Robuvit® metabolites appear to affect ribosome, cell cycle, and spliceosome pathways. However, these cellular effects are difficult to compare to actual human, clinical models.

Robuvit® extract concentrates water-soluble components of the wood (defined as ellagitannins) also found in wine that have been resting in oak barrels. Flavors are imported into the wine from the wood as it ages in oak barrels. The use of oak has been prevalent in winemaking for centuries. These substances derived from oak wood are considered completely safe. Wine in the barrel acquires different types of tannins. This specific supplement from oak wood is specified to contain in its PS supplement at least 20% of roburins (A, B, C, D and E) and grandinin. Both components belong to the group of hydrolyzable tannins (also defined ellagitannins).

Clinical investigations in healthy volunteers and patients in different clinical conditions have preliminarily shown an increased antioxidant capacity of the blood after supplementation. Also, a significant decrease in peripheral edema after supplementation with Robuvit® has been observed. Lymphatic edema (mainly primary lymphedema and lymphedema secondary to surgery or radiotherapy) is specifically affected.

The most important hydrolyzable tannins included in Robuvit® may be effective — the supplement is under evaluation — in different preclinical and clinical conditions (associated with chronic inflammation) as they have a basic anti-inflammatory action. The product is active at a dosage between 100 and 300 mg. The strong antioxidant efficacy of Robuvit® has been tested in healthy volunteers (improving oxidative stress), in patients with hepatic failure, with good results on hepatic functional values. Data from this pilot, supplement registry study indicate a significant protective activity of Robuvit®, associated with a very good safety profile, in patients with temporary hepatic failure. The activity of Robuvit® seems to be mediated by its combined antioxidant and anti-inflammatory activity.

Robuvit® has been also effective in the management of subjects with chronic fatigue syndrome and increased oxidative stress. These subjects improved with Robuvit® supplementation in comparison with untreated controls. No side effects have been observed during or after Robuvit® supplementation so far. Robuvit® is still in development, and it could be considered the first PS supplement of this kind.

S-adenosyl-L-methionine

S-adenosyl-L-methionine (SAM) is a derivative of methionine and a cofactor for multiple synthetic pathways. It is produced naturally in the body and manufactured synthetically in several PS supplement forms. It is a common cosubstrate involved in methyl group transfers.

SAM was discovered in Italy by G. L. Cantoni in 1952. It is produced from adenosine triphosphate (ATP) and methionine by methionine adenosyltransferase. Transmethylation, transsulfuration, and aminopropylation are the metabolic pathways that use SAM. These anabolic reactions occur anywhere in the body, but most SAM is produced and consumed in the liver.

Claims

SAM is said to be effective for treatment of depression, OA and liver disorders, but scientific studies so far do not confirm this claim. More research is needed to verify its clinical efficacy. Some research, including clinical trials, indicated that SAM used on a regular basis may help in the management of depression; SAM may have some effects in the treatment of liver diseases and may help in the chronic management of pain in patients with OA.

The Dietary Supplement Health and Education Act (1994) allows the distribution of SAM as a supplement by passing the regulatory requirements for drugs (by the FDA). When a series of studies found evidence of abnormally low levels of endogenous SAM that may have a role in the evolution of Alzheimer's disease, SAM was considered to have therapeutic potential in this field. However, further research has indicated this effect is likely due to vitamin B_{12} deficiencies, which cause neurological alterations (due to the inability to conduct 1-carbon transfers with folate in the absence of vitamin B_{12}). Very low levels of SAM have been found in the cerebrospinal fluid and in other brain regions in Alzheimer's disease patients. However, this clinical line of research is almost impossible to define and follow due to costs, prolonged times and variability of clinical patterns.

Adverse effects

No serious adverse effects have been reported. SAM is contraindicated in patients with bipolar disorder because SAM can precipitate manic episodes. GI disorder, dyspepsia and anxiety can occur with SAM supplements. Long-term effects are unknown. SAM is a weak DNA-alkylating agent. When used with some drugs, it may increase the risk of serotonin syndrome, a potentially dangerous condition caused by having too much serotonin. These drugs include dextromethorphan (Robitussin®), meperidine (Demerol®), pentazocine (Talwin®), and tramadol (Ultram®). SAM may also interact with antidepressant medications increasing the potential for their side effects and reduce the effectiveness of levodopa for Parkinson's disease.

Saw palmetto

The Mayans drank saw palmetto (SP) as a tonic, and the Seminoles used the berries as an expectorant and antiseptic. The extract of SP is produced from the fruit of *Serenoa repens* rich in fatty acids and phytosterols. PS supplements have been used to treat a variety of conditions, mostly benign prostatic hyperplasia (BPH). Recent clinical trials found the extract to be marginally more effective than placebo for BPH. However, the *Merck Manual* clearly indicates SP as an effective supplement for BPH (Figure 21).

Only berries from SP contain the plant's active ingredients in reasonable quantities. The active ingredients (possibly fatty acids) are still unidentified, but they appear to inhibit 3a-reductase opposing the conversion

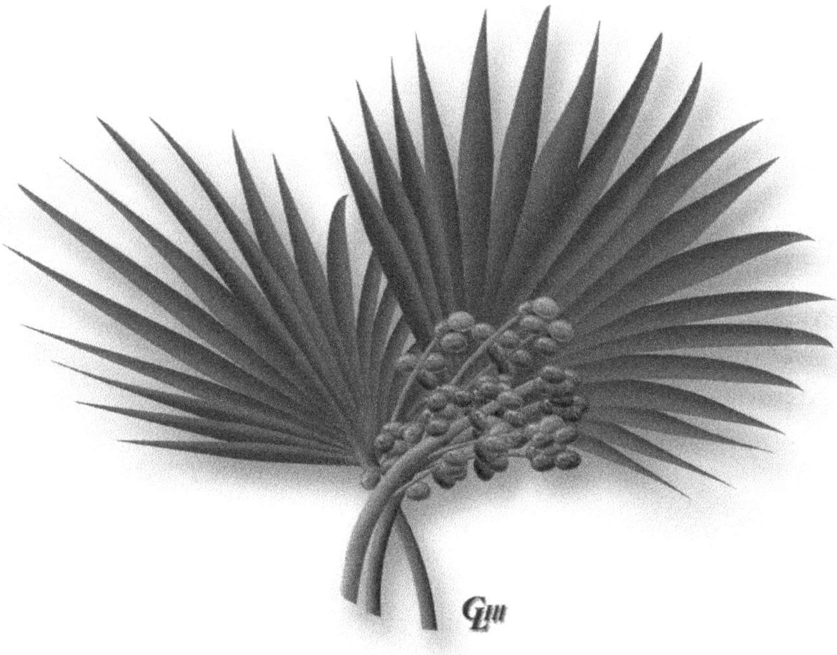

Figure 21: Saw palmetto.

of testosterone to dihydrotestosterone. PS supplements used in recent studies are made with hexane extracts of SP berries including which are 80–90% essential fatty acids and phytosterols.

Claims

Strong scientific evidence supports use of SP PS supplements to treat symptoms of BPH (e.g., frequent urination, dysuria, etc.). Clinical evidence suggests that it may reverse — at least partially — in time the hyperplasia. But some large studies did not show any benefit on the evolution of hyperplasia.

There are claims that SP supplements may increase sperm production, breast size or sexual vigor — in younger men — but these results are basically unproven. For PS supplements, the dose is 320 mg once a day or 160 mg bid. Generally, around 2 months' time is needed to detect significant improvements in signs/symptoms in most patients. At the moment, SP extract and supplements are the most popular "plant-derived" treatment for BPH.

Adverse effects

Headache and diarrhea may occur in some subjects. β-Sitosterol, a chemical present in SP extract, is chemically similar to cholesterol. High levels of sitosterol concentrations in blood have correlated with increased severity of heart disease in men who previously suffered heart attacks. No other serious adverse effects have been reported so far. SP supplements may interact with estrogen; thus, women who are pregnant or who may become pregnant should not take it.

SP extracts can theoretically slow down clotting, leading to increased bleeding time before and after surgery. Patients taking SP may have increased bleeding time during surgery. The bleeding time returns to normal after the patient stops supplementation. The use of SP supplements should also be stopped at least two weeks before a scheduled surgical procedure. Also, effects on the coagulation and aggregation can be seen in association with antiplatelets agents.

Sophora japonica

Styphnolobium japonicum (医疗中心), the pagoda tree (*Sophora japonica*), is a species of tree in the subfamily Faboideae of the pea family Fabaceae. It has abortifacient, antibacterial, anticholesterolemic, anti-inflammatory, antispasmodic, diuretic, emetic, emollient, febrifuge, hypotensive, purgative, styptic and tonic properties. *Styphnolobium japonicum* contains the isoflavone glycoside sophoricoside (Figure 22).

The Chinese name for the tree (槐) is composed of the word 木 ("wood") and 鬼 ("demon"). It appears that the presence of this tree keeps away other plants by different poisonous substances. It has been safely and effectively used in several PS supplements for the treatment of CVI and VV and diabetic microangiopathy (Venoruton®, Novartis).

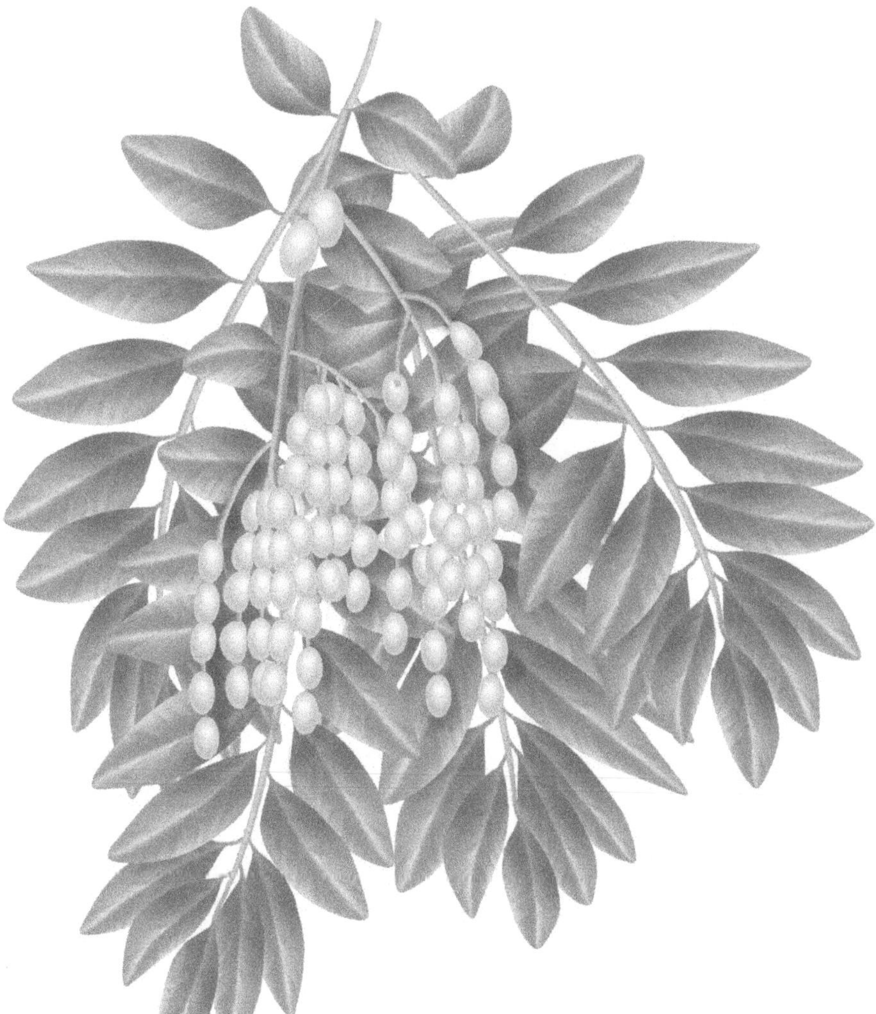

Figure 22: *Sophora japonica.*

St. John's wort

St. John's wort (SJW, *Hypericum perforatum*) is a flowering plant species of the genus *Hypericum*. It is a medicinal herb with significant antidepressant properties and potential antibacterial and anti-inflammatory properties.

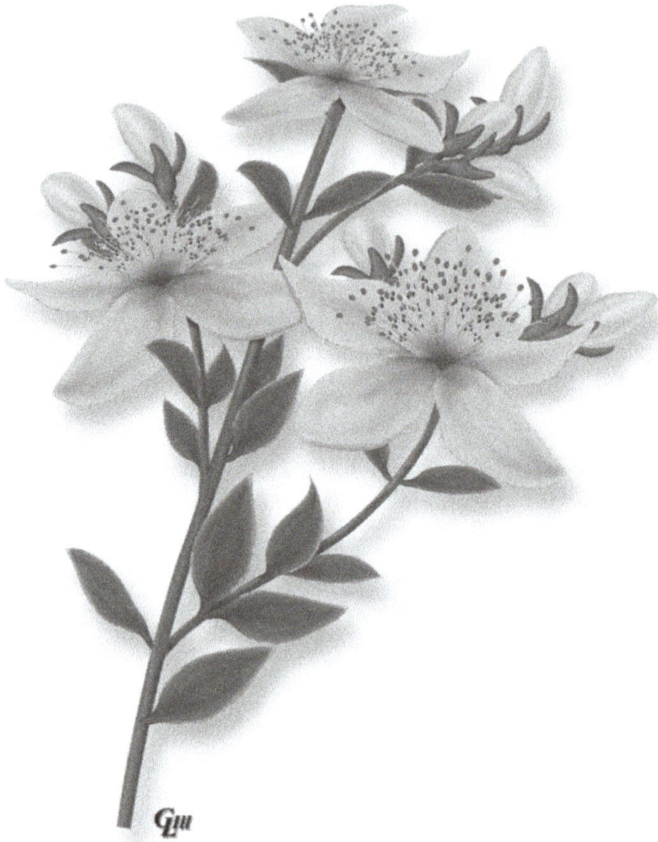

Figure 23: St. John's wort.

Extracts of SJW can be used as a treatment for depression. SJW flowers contain its biologically active ingredients hypericin and hyperforin. SJW may increase central nervous system serotonin, and in very high doses, it acts like an MAOI (Figure 23).

Claims

Study findings are variable, but SJW PS supplements may be used by patients with mild to moderate depression who have no suicidal tendency. However, a large study found SJW ineffective in treating major depression. The dose is 300–600 mg per os, once a day of a PS supplement's preparation (0.2–0.3% hypericin to 1–4% hyperforin).

SJW may also be useful in treating HIV infection, but there are proven adverse interactions with protease inhibitors and nonnucleoside reverse transcriptase inhibitors (NNRTIs). A small study indicated that SJW supplements (standardized to hypericin but not to hyperforin) were not effective in relieving symptoms of attention-deficit hyperactivity disorder in children.

SJW has shown some possible actions in Parkinson's disease indicating that SJW has antioxidant active ingredients that may reduce the neuronal degeneration caused by the disease. Hypericin and pseudohypericin have shown both antiviral and antibacterial activities. These molecules bind nonspecifically to viral and cellular membranes and can result in photooxidation of the pathogens, eventually killing them.

Adverse effects

Minor effects include photosensitivity, dry mouth, constipation, dizziness, confusion, and more important side effects may include manic manifestations (in patients with bipolar disorder). SJW should not be used in pregnant women. Potential adverse interactions may occur with cyclosporine, digoxin, iron supplements, MAOIs, NNRTIs, oral contraceptives, protease inhibitors, SSRIs, tricyclic antidepressants and anticoagulants.

Valerian

Valerian (*Valeriana officinalis)* (Caprifoliaceae) is a perennial flowering plant with heads of sweetly scented pink or white flowers that bloom in the summer months. Valerian flower extracts were used as a perfume. Valerian's root and rhizomes (underground stems) contain its active ingredients, including valepotriates and pungent odiferous oils. Crude extract of the root is often sold in the form of capsules. Valerian root has sedative and anxiolytic effects. It can also be classified as a drug, since its consumption produces a sedative or medicinal effect, while it is not exclusively a type of food. These effects are possibly mediated through the gamma-aminobutyric acid (GABA) receptor. The amino acid valine is named after the name of the plant (Figure 24).

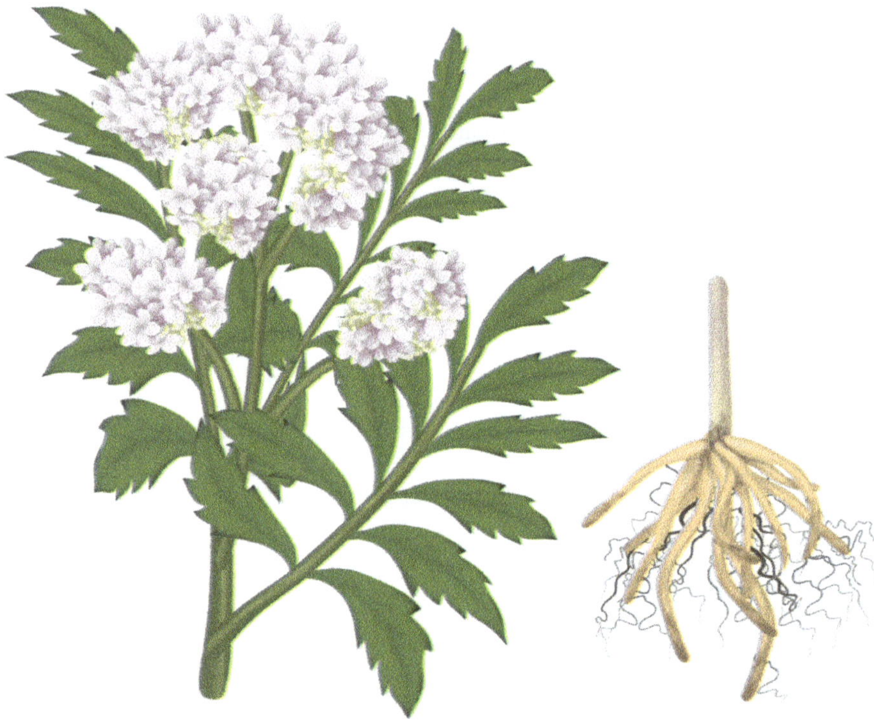

Figure 24: Valerian.

Known compounds detected in valerian that may contribute to its method of action are as follows:

- alkaloids: actinidine, chatinine, shyanthine, valerianine and valerine,
- isovaleramide may be created in the extraction process,
- GABA,
- isovaleric acid,
- iridoids, including valepotriates: isovaltrate and valtrate,
- sesquiterpenes (contained in the volatile oil): valerenic acid, hydroxy-valerenic acid and acetoxyvalerenic acid,
- flavanones: hesperidin, 6-methylapigenin and linarin.

Claims

Valerian is generally used as a weak, reliable and safe sedative and as a to-get-sleep aid. In several studies, valerian improved sleep quality and shortened the time needed to fall asleep. However, these observations are very difficult to evaluate and quantify; there is insufficient clinical experience (but this is not really a clinical problem) to confirm whether valerian is effective for insomnia. For mild nonclinical problems, it could be a mildly effective and safe solution.

Some people take valerian for headaches, even depression, irregular heartbeat, anxiety or trembling linked to some form of stress. There is not enough evidence to determine whether valerian may work for these conditions. Valerian is usually — as extract or PS supplement — used for short periods of time (4–6 weeks); most studies and experience suggest that it is generally safe.

Adverse effects

Valerian may theoretically prolong the effect of other sedatives (e.g., barbiturates) and — always in theory — affect driving or other activities requiring alertness. It may be more effective in subjects using antihistamine drugs. A meta-analysis ("How can you make a meta-analysis with different products, administrations and dosages?") published in 2006 in the *American Journal of Medicine* concluded that available evidence indicate that valerian might improve sleep quality without producing side effects.

How you assess sleep quality is a real issue. Most effects could be individually based. An article in the *Medical Science Monitor* indicated that "... based on cellular and animal (again what kind of animal model can you use for getting sleep?) studies as well as human clinical (clinical?) trials there is a role for valerian (including root extract) as useful alternatives in the management of stress and anxiety". Another systematic review in the journal *Sleep Medicine Review* (2007) indicated that valerian is safe but not clinically (clinically?) effective for insomnia.

Actually, valerian is a very good model to discuss some aspects of this field. Many patented drugs have less evidence than most PS supplements for efficacy and definitely much lower levels of safety and tolerability. For valerian, there is a possible very important, individual component that should be considered and respected.

Zinc

The naturally occurring mineral zinc is required in small quantities in multiple metabolic pathways. Dietary sources include oysters, beef and fortified cereals. Zinc is an essential mineral of "exceptional biologic and public health importance". Zinc deficiency affects about two billion people in the developing world and is associated with many diseases. In children, it causes growth retardation, delayed sexual maturation, infection susceptibility and diarrhea, contributing to the death of about 800,000 children worldwide per year.

Enzymes with a zinc atom in the reactive center are widespread in biochemistry, such as alcohol dehydrogenase in humans. Consumption of excess zinc can cause ataxia, lethargy and copper deficiency. Zinc deficiency has been associated with major depressive disorder (MDD), and zinc supplements may be an effective treatment.

Claims

Some experts believe that when taken soon after cold symptoms develop, zinc (used as zinc gluconate or acetate lozenges) may shorten the course of the common cold. Studies are limited — as for any nonpatentable product — but zinc even with a limited effect, occurring when it is taken very soon after cold symptoms develop, may reduce the global effect of cold. Reduction of just 1 day in the course of cold may reduce the number of days of diseases in millions of patients with a significant reduction in health costs.

There is stronger evidence that in developing countries, supplements containing zinc 20 mg and iron taken once a week reduce mortality in infants who have diarrhea and respiratory infection. There is also strong evidence that zinc supplements containing 80 mg and antioxidants once a day slow progression of moderate to severe atrophic (dry form) age-related maculopathy in elderly people. Basically, zinc is too cheap to be good.

Adverse effects

Zinc is generally considered safe, but toxicity can develop if high doses are used. Common adverse effects of zinc lozenges include nausea, vomiting, diarrhea, mouth irritation, mouth sores and bad metallic taste. Zinc is a trace metal and can remove other necessary metals from the body; therefore, zinc lozenges should not be taken for more than 3 weeks. Some zinc sprays may cause nose and throat irritation. The effects of certain antibiotics may be altered and decreased by the consumption of zinc supplements.

3

PS Supplements in Different Clinical Conditions

Cardiovascular disease

In cardiovascular disease, PS supplements can be used in preclinical and preventive applications, in borderline problems (hypertension, hyperlipidemia) and in clinical conditions. Such supplements may be used for long periods of time and, very often, in concomitance with other products (i.e., antiplatelet agents or anticoagulants, antihypertensives, etc.), so safety in the use of these supplements is essential.

A negative interaction with antiplatelet agents has been considered, but this is mainly theoretical and more or less irrelevant from a clinical point of view. The interaction with anticoagulants is taken more seriously as it is possible that potentially severe clinical problems are associated with decreased clotting and increased hemorrhage or bleeding tendency or an increase in clotting that may lead to thrombosis.

Any supplement that could be used by patients or physicians for any cardiovascular condition (or in any patient with cardiovascular problems requiring medical treatment) should be safe. It should be tested for potential thrombogenicity or for its facilitation activity upon bleeding or anticoagulation. There are several claims about products that may help to decrease *total lipids*, but to date, only green tea and FO are considered to be of use in any significant way, based upon recent studies.

Chromium picolinate and garlic supplements decrease *triglyceride* levels (in some patients) but not without further dietary action. *HDL increase* has been shown in studies with garlic and ginseng supplements. *Heart failure* has been improved with CoQ10 supplementation. CoQ10 appears also useful to fight anthracycline. CoQ10 is generally decreased in a number of patients using statins and some cholesterol-lowering drugs. The decrease in CoQ10 in tissues (including myocardium) is associated with muscular pain and fatigue and with possible heart failure. Restoring normal CoQ10 levels may be essential in decreasing mortality in patients using statins for a long period of time.

Blood pressure and atherosclerosis

Blood pressure has been shown to improve with FO PS supplements. Borderline hypertensive patients had significant benefits by being supplemented with Pycnogenol® in a recent specific study on otherwise healthy borderline hypertensives, with a grape seed PS supplement. A global (small) reduction in *lipids* has been suggested with green tea. However, the quantity of reduction is difficult to define and it is probably minimal from a clinical point of view. Definitely, one green tea (Camellia) PS supplement improves blood pressure in borderline subjects with metabolic syndrome, including increased blood pressure.

In terms of sheer numbers and complexity, *atherosclerosis* is the real challenge in cardiovascular disease. It is the mother of all other cardiovascular problems. The control and treatment of atherosclerosis is essential for the management of most cardiovascular patients. No single treatment for atherosclerosis is available, this being a result of its multifactorial and multifaceted characterization. The tendency toward irregular growth of plaques in the arteries is at least almost always at hemodynamically important points (i.e., bifurcations of the carotid and coronary arteries, in low shear stress parts of the arterial segments), and so this can be monitored and treated, if not eradicated.

Atherosclerosis, like many diseases, is age related, and it is difficult to manage or treat ageing. Atherosclerosis is the most diffuse and demanding of age-related diseases, with its attendant costs, complications and complexity of interrelated problems. There is evidence that in subjects with increased plasmatic oxidative stress ("oxstress"), the genesis, evolution and progression of plaques is faster. This is why antioxidants are considered useful to stop progression.

A recent study indicated that the combination Pycnogenol® + CA decreases the growth of atherosclerotic plaques (in the carotid, aorta and femoral arteries and very possibly, at coronary level) independently from a reduction in the major risk factors. Such studies last years and require large numbers of patients. Studies also indicate that lipids enter the arterial wall in the presence of higher oxidative stress and that plaques grow faster in the presence of oxidative stress. The combination CA + Pycnogenol® appears to reduce the irregular deposition of collagen in atherosclerotic plaques reducing their progression and controlling the passage to symptomatic stages; this happens in concomitance with the control of altered (increased) oxstress.

A significant number of subjects may remain asymptomatic (the plaques do not grow to become clinically important) for years. The use of a concomitant antiplatelet agent is facilitated in its action by Pycnogenol® which also has an intrinsic antiplatelet action. A small atherosclerotic plaque includes a universe of life conditions, diseases and diseased conditions leading to such complexity that it will take ages to define and stop. At the moment, a more regular incorporation of collagen into the plaque, controlling inflammation and oxstress, seems a very good start to stop the progression of atherosclerosis and a significant, safe and easy clinical option to offer to many patients.

Microcirculation

Microcirculation changes (e.g., in diabetic microangiopathy or vasospastic disorders) may be obtained with Pycnogenol® and ginkgo. Results may be clinically important in most individuals. Curcumin (Meriva®) may stop the progression of diabetic microangiopathy — and possibly that of retinopathy — in longer studies. *Microcirculation studies are key to the evaluation of most modern PS supplements and their clinical effects.* One recent study shows that *endothelial dysfunction* may be improved with Pycnogenol® and FO, but the results are clinically difficult to evaluate. One study showed endothelial function was improved with Pycnogenol®

in subjects with severe coronary problems. However, endothelial dysfunction is an early observation in the development of atherosclerosis (i.e., in subjects without plaques), and it is more a risk condition than a real disease that may require treatment.

Often the risk factor *causing* endothelial dysfunction (i.e., hypertension, hypercholesterolemia) should be clinically addressed in the first place. The "treatment" of endothelial dysfunction — which is not a disease — should not be a main target but may be an accessory in the evaluation of PS supplements. The risk of *myocardial infarction* (MI) has been reduced in some studies with FO. Also, recurrence of MI may be reduced using proper management and FO. *Arrhythmia* can be also controlled with FO in some patients or controlled with valerian.

Reduction of caloric load and lipid absorption, a metabolic target rather than a cardiovascular one, seems a logical step in the control of atherosclerosis. But it is not considered a real cardiovascular treatment. However, it is noted that Camellia, the green tea PS supplement, appears to control *all lipids* in borderline metabolic syndrome. Effects on peripheral vascular disease (associated with claudication) have previously been shown with ginkgo PS supplements.

Venous disease

Both signs and symptoms associated with varicose veins and CVI are effectively and safely treated even for long periods with Pycnogenol®, which is the most powerful compound usable in venous disease. *Sophora japonica* is present as an essential component in one of the leading products used for venous disease (Venoruton®, Novartis), and it is highly effective and safe. Grape leaf supplements and supplements including CA are also used. *Centella* is seen to be more effective in advanced stages, and in healing venous ulcers.

Pycnogenol® has also been effectively used to heal venous ulcers, even in topical formulations. The main action of Pycnogenol® is in its ability to control edema at capillary level in venous hypertensive microangiopathy. Diabetic and venous microangiopathy are both "high-perfusion" microangiopathies and are associated to edema. Edema control at capillary level improves nutrition and perfusion and promotes healing with similar mechanisms.

Lymphatic disease

At the moment, there is no specific treatment for primary lymphedema. Edema in lymphatic patients is characterized by a high level of proteins in the interstitial fluid. Primary lymphedema is very rare and no significant company has invested in a problems that is limited. Postsurgical or postradiotherapy lymphedema is a common observation that requires a complex of treatments. The french oak wood PS supplement Robuvit® has recently shown an important action in patients with primary lymphedema controlling signs and symptoms. More studies are in progress. *Sophora japonica* may also be useful.

Supplements, thrombosis and rethrombosis prevention, thrombogenicity

Nattokinase and Pycnogenol® in combination are found in an antithrombotic product (Flite Tabs®) that has been tested in long flights with good results (however, more subjects are needed). Pycnogenol® is being used in open registry studies on recurrent DVT and in retinal thrombosis (to prevent further episodes) with results that are better than aspirin (<5% recurrence at 5 y). Pycnogenol® also appears to decrease the occurrence of postthrombotic syndrome, mainly by controlling postthrombotic edema. Specific studies on the efficacy and potential clinical value of Pycnogenol® as an antithrombotic agent are in progress.

Joints and bones

Arthrosis and arthritis

There are two types of problems due to osteoarthritis (OA). Firstly, an inflammatory process may be present and active and may be the main cause of the arthrosis. Further, a mainly degenerative process (i.e., due to excessive weight on the knee) may cause comparable or concomitant OA problems. The aim of treatments with PS supplements is to decrease pain and stiffness making the patients able to walk and regain some or all normal functions again.

OA can be effectively treated with black cohosh PS supplement which is known to improve symptoms. Chondroitin sulfate (CS) is also effective, but the positive effects may be minimal in some subjects if used as a single treatment. The combination of *chondroitin with glucosamine* makes most combination supplements effective, well tolerated and practical and may allow many of these patients to avoid long periods of use of NSAIDs, with many potential consequences in costs and side effects.

PS supplements with green tea, S-adenosyl-L-methionine, curcumin and Pycnogenol® have been used to successfully reduce pain and inflammation. The effects of treatments may be very individual. In more severe phases with strong inflammation and pain, other "heavier" treatments may be needed, but in "remission" periods, most supplements are safe, effective, well tolerated and cost effective. The short-term target could be improving signs and symptoms, and the long-term target, if possible, could be rebuilding some of the damaged cartilage, restoring the cartilage to stages closer to its initial functional physiology and morphology.

Improving joint mobility, stiffness, walking distance without pain with PS supplements allows a significant reduction in the need for costly, time-consuming "conventional" management methods (i.e., physiotherapy, rehabilitation and hospital admission). New PS products including Meriva® (curcumin), *Boswellia* and Pycnogenol® have been shown to improve the Karnofsky scale (the global functional ability of patients) and the WOMAC score (specifically devised to study OA with its signs and symptoms) even delaying the need for surgery in some patients. Feverfew supplements have also been used. The treatments with supplements should be adapted to each single patient and all the factors aggravating the clinical picture (e.g., excessive weight, a sedentary life) should also be aggressively corrected.

Rheumatoid arthritis and conditions with a very strong inflammatory component have been successfully treated with black cohosh PS supplements. A recent study shows that Pycnogenol® lowers C-reactive protein and oxidative stress in symptomatic patients with OA. OA management is one of the most important fields of application for supplements and should be well known by all physicians and practitioners dealing with these patients.

Menopausal transition

Signs and symptoms could be controlled on a very individual basis using black cohosh supplements, green tea and Pycnogenol®. Menopause is not a disease, but it certainly does negatively affect a great many women. Studies with Pycnogenol® show very good effects in pre- and postmenopausal women and during the menopausal transition. Other symptoms like vaginal dryness and small infections, particularly in diabetic menopausal women were positively affected by a specific PS supplement (Lady Prelox®) including Pycnogenol®, Rosvita®, L-arginine and L-citrulline.

Menstrual symptoms are attenuated (on an individual basis) by black cohosh, feverfew and Pycnogenol®. Estrogenic effects can be obtained with ginseng, but there are only a limited number of case studies so far. Some recurrent vaginal infections could be treated with goldenseal supplements. The many aspects of the functional and physiological sexual life of women (including the menopausal transition) should be better explored in all their phases. This should become a very significant field of action for many supplements.

New supplements (including ferula) are in advanced phases of development. Most signs and symptoms are merely an expression of physiology rather than a pathology and may benefit from "mild–soft" management with supplements, leaving drugs for more severe, debilitating pathological conditions.

Inflammation

Inflammation is a significant component of most pathological processes that require treatment when excessive and out of control. Chamomile and ginger supplements may reduce both local and systemic mild inflammatory processes without using more significant, dangerous and costly drugs that may cause side effects. Some "bark steroids" may have a profile comparable to corticosteroids on inflammation but with a weaker physiological action with a less dangerous pattern and frequency of side effects (i.e., *Boswellia*, Pycnogenol®, curcumin) and should be considered instead of corticosteroid (for instance, in remission phases when the full action of corticosteroids is not needed).

Fever

Fever is one of the most common signs and should always be managed with great attention. Chamomile and cranberry PS supplements may help. It is possible that other supplements could be used, but this field requires research.

Gastrointestinal and hepatic diseases

This is another field of great interest for PS supplements with many effective products available. Stomach cramps may benefit from chamomile. Signs of indigestion have also been treated with chamomile and goldenseal supplements, and gastritis (even ulcers in the past) has been treated with chamomile and licorice, either in their natural forms or as supplements. Vomiting and nausea (including motion sickness and pregnancy) may be relieved by ginger supplements. Symptoms of diarrhea can be mitigated with goldenseal supplements.

Acute mild–moderate hepatitis associated to drug treatments or alcohol (and marginally even some cases of cirrhosis) can be positively affected with milk thistle (MT) supplements, with Robuvit® (as shown in two recent studies) and by S-adenosyl-L-methionine. Both Liverubin® (Alchem) and Robuvit® were effective in improving enzyme patterns (normalizing bilirubin and improving albumin) in a matter of weeks with a very good safety profile, essential in these patients.

In these cases (there is no established drug or treatment for moderate hepatitis of this kind), the physician should not add the damage potentially caused by a treatment to an already established hepatic failure that may precipitate in case of further damage. Mushroom poisoning — very dangerous and fast in its evolution — could benefit from high-dosage MT supplements. However, the number of cases is very limited and the patients are never "standard" cases. There is a very large variability of clinical conditions.

Asthma

Feverfew has been used in asthma, and it could be effective on an individual basis (the patient may try the supplement and judge whether it is effective for his/her situation or not). Pycnogenol® has been also used in stable, otherwise healthy patients, with good functional results and improvements in signs and symptoms. A study has also indicated that Pycnogenol® may have a histamine-controlling effect that needs to be evaluated in larger clinical studies.

Tracheal burning or irritation, sore throat and other symptoms due to involvement of the upper respiratory tract can be relieved by ginger supplements and expectorant including licorice. A specific product (PhytoRelief-CC®) containing ginger and pomegranate may be effective both for treatment and control and for prevention of viral infections. Studies are in progress.

Weight loss

Whilst weight loss is *not a clinical problem* by itself and is not a disease, there is certainly a regularly trending interest in methods of weight control. Modern life is now much more sedentary than it was previously and affects many more people, thus causing a global increase in average weight, which has effects on health and optimum bodily function.

Chromium picolinate has been used to reduce body fat and for the metabolic control of risk factors: it may increase insulin function. The supplementation does not help diabetics, and the effects on body composition may be minimal. Camellia (a PS green tea supplement) has been effectively used in subjects with borderline metabolic syndrome with good results in limited studies and absolute safety and tolerability. Pycnogenol® also helps in borderline metabolic syndrome and it had been used with significant results in specific subjects with an inflammatory component (i.e., increased C-reactive protein) and/or increased oxidative stress.

Weight loss cannot be achieved with drugs. There are too many components. Eating smaller portions, eating less junk food and exercising is still the main key to weight loss. But we need to have a double-blind study to show this concept and an endorsement from Cochrane.

Immune stimulation

This is not a clinical condition or a disease, unless we include subjects with immunodepression caused by severe problems, e.g., HIV, radio- or chemotherapy. When using supplements, the meaning of "immune stimulation" is related more to the efficiency of a defense system against viral aggression (i.e., flu or cold). CoQ10 supplements, *Echinacea* and ginseng have shown the capacity to increase resistance to minor viral infections (cold or flu). The idea that stimulating the immune system may prevent cancer is a really dreamy concept but has never yet been properly shown in a clinical setting or study.

Colds and flu are the most frequent diseases, and a prevention method could be very important. Supplements including *Echinacea* or ginseng or PS supplements with goldenseal have been shown to be effective in reducing the duration (and severity) of colds; zinc has been studied in several clinical experiences and appears to reduce the duration of cold episodes.

Adding vitamin C seems to have a minimal effect. It is more likely that vitamin C should be used during periods of time *before* an episode to have any effect. The number of subjects with flu or cold, the number of tracheal-bronco-pulmonary complications due to severe flu (including hospital admission, particularly in older, higher-risk subjects) has been reduced using colostrum. Colostrum appeared more effective than the antiflu vaccination and is considered to be very safe. It is clear that very large studies are needed for this kind of evaluation.

Products should always be used considering context, the basic health of the subject to be supplemented, and results should be evaluated on an individual basis. Even shortening a flu or cold episode by a single day each time would enormously decrease medical costs and problems.

Kidney and urinary infections

Cranberry has been successfully used and is recommended for common, mild–moderate and recurrent urinary tract infections (UTIs). The use of cranberry PS supplements is effective in reducing not only the colonization by most common bacteria but also the inflammation after a real infection is completely treated and there are no longer detectable bacteria in the urine.

Cranberry can also be used during the postcatheterization period when a mix of mild inflammation and infection may persist and cause symptoms. Cranberry is particularly effective in recurrent small infections in healthy subjects (particularly in women). A severe infection in patients with other clinical problems should be aggressively treated with the appropriate antibiotic. The administration of cranberry should be continued for some 60 d.

Cranberry has no side effect, but it promotes acidity in urine and may therefore promote the formation of uric acid kidney stones in predisposed individuals. Theoretically it may interact with anticoagulants. Concerning the kidney, *cyclosporine nephrotoxicity* — and possibly other kinds of nephrotoxicity — has been shown to be attenuated with FO supplements and with ginkgo.

Benign prostatic hypertrophy (BPH)

In different types of formulation, saw palmetto (SP) has been shown to be effective in the management of BPH. It is used as a significant treatment and is competitive with "standard" treatments. SP has very few side effects (possibly diarrhea or headache on an individual basis) and could be an important choice for starting a treatment in the case of initial symptoms of BPH or when drugs are not tolerated or have caused the side effect of intolerance.

The complex *Echinacea* + SP in a PS supplement appears to be more effective than SP alone. Patients may start with SP supplement and evaluate for themselves whether the efficacy of the treatment is suitable for them. It is possible that SP may be effective on an individual basis and also that some subjects may be less responsive to the supplement.

Eyes

Creatine administration can help positively with gyrate atrophy of the choroid and retina. This is a very specialized application of creatine and requires specific competence. Creatine can also be effective in age-related maculopathy. The retinal microcirculation may be affected by ginkgo (improving flow) and Pycnogenol® (with a specific activity on edema control and also improving retinal flow). The evolution of diabetic micro-angiopathy (at retinal level) can be improved in longer periods using curcumin (Meriva®).

A specific combination (Mirtogenol®) has been recently developed for the microcirculation of the eye. This supplement is a combination of standardized bilberry extract (from fresh fruit of *Vaccinium myrtillus*, called Mirtoselect®) and Pycnogenol®. Improving optical microcirculation may also be effective (in selected patients) in reducing ocular pressure. The optic nerve is damaged by higher intraocular pressures; the decrease in the blood flow to the optic nerve makes this nerve susceptible to the damage induced by the high levels of intraocular pressure. However, more studies are needed in a larger number of subjects.

Neurology

Supplementation in the field of neurology has so far been disappointing (although the same could be said for most drug treatments). However, this is a large and interesting field, and there is much to research.

The blood–brain barrier (BBB) is a highly selective permeability barrier. It separates the circulating blood in capillaries from the brain extracellular fluid (BECF) in the central nervous system (CNS). The BBB is a structure based on capillary endothelial cells, connected by tight junctions with an extremely high electrical resistance. The BBB allows the selective passage of water, some gases and lipid-soluble molecules (by passive diffusion).

Selective transport of molecules (using energy) is used for glucose, amino acids and elements that are essential for the functions of the neural network. The BBB selectively prevents the passage of lipophilic, potential neurotoxins (by an active transport mechanism mediated by P-glycoprotein). Astrocytes are necessary for the BBB. A small number of regions and areas in the brain, including the circumventricular organs (CVOs), do not have a BBB.

Morphologically, the BBB is situated around capillaries and includes tight junctions around the capillaries which do not exist in the normal distal circulation. Endothelial cells restrict the diffusion of microscopic objects (e.g., bacteria) and large or hydrophilic molecules into the cerebrospinal fluid (CSF) but allow the diffusion of small hydrophobic molecules (O_2, CO_2, hormones). Many supplements do not reach the BBB, and most do not pass it. Therefore, experiences are limited and disappointing. There is some evidence of an efficacy of creatine in *Parkinson's* disease.

DHEA has been evaluated in *mood disorders* with some results. *Insomnia and sleep disorders* are improved by DHEA, chamomile supplements, melatonin and valerian but on an individual basis. In *Alzheimer's disease*, DHEA has been used with contrasting results (most treatments do not work in this condition, which means it is an increasingly important field of study). Ginkgo supplements may help subjects with *dementia*. The problem is that ginkgo will improve the arterial flow and microcirculation in the brain, but this does not mean that the cerebral and neurological functions are improved. *Migraine* has been treated with some success (individual basis) with feverfew supplements.

Problems related to *jet lag* (sleep disorders, attention deficits, desynchronization, decreased mental performance, etc.) have been improved with melatonin (as melatonin may improve sleep and rest). Studies with Pycnogenol® indicate that most jet-lag-related problems may be due to a minimal accumulation of fluid in the brain (similar to that which occurs in the lower limbs). The control of edema may be effective in preventing both cerebral and leg edema (fluid accumulation during long flights) and in the restoration of normal cerebral function. The effect has been noted to be more evident in subjects using antihypertensive drugs, who are particularly prone to edema. Jet lag is an important model (it is not a disease) showing that the regulation of water — possibly causing edema — out of the BBB may actually improve cerebral functions.

Depression (which is a wide definition of many differing conditions) has been positively affected, in some subjects, with S-adenosyl-L-methionine and with supplements of St. John's wort. Mild *anxiety* (also considered to include a wide range of clinical and subclinical conditions) may be effectively and safely treated with such sedative supplements as chamomile and valerian.

Wound healing

Several products can be used for wound healing: *Echinacea* supplements have shown significant effects; also Pycnogenol® and CA have been effectively used for ulcers (both venous due to deep venous insufficiency (DVI) and diabetic ulcers due to microangiopathy). CA also reduced the formation of cheloids (i.e., in children after burns) and irregular cicatrization.

Platelet aggregation

Several supplements claim some activity of platelet aggregation. Very often, the effect is not clinically relevant, and it is not dangerous. Feverfew and S-adenosyl-L-methionine may alter platelet function. Pycnogenol® studies indicate an antiplatelet action that may be synergic with other antiplatelet agents (i.e., aspirin) and may be of clinical interest and value.

Diabetes

As such, diabetes *per se* does not seem affected by most supplements, but some products may either improve diabetic control or make the control of diabetes more difficult or interfere with the many treatments used by diabetics. Ginseng supplements may have a significant action on diabetes, but it needs to be evaluated in larger studies.

Generally, the field of PS supplements should receive more attention — and more targeted research — for this diffuse and challenging condition leading to so many complications and preventable deaths. However, the push of many big pharma companies in this field — often practically working as a cartel — make it almost impossible or at least not competitive enough to enable entry into this huge market by smaller companies with potentially interesting products. Also, diabetics constitute a "poor" market. Most diabetics in most National Health (NH) systems receive all their medications for free, any drug or product, and they are not motivated or accustomed to spending money on such things as PS supplements.

Antimicrobial activity

The activity of PS supplements (excluding cranberry with its high specificity for UTI) is not really usable for clinical applications. The theoretic antimicrobic activity of several products has a minimal clinical value.

Tinnitus

It is possible that tinnitus could be affected by ginkgo supplements and by Pycnogenol®. However, ginkgo may work only on tinnitus with a significant vascular component (improving the microcirculation) and therefore is effective only on tinnitus of vascular origin. Pycnogenol® is also effective on the microcirculation and may help reduce edema in a region with minimal vein drainage and no lymphatic component. Therefore, alteration in the microcirculation (i.e., vasospasm, reduced flow) or cochlear edema should be present before considering the use of the supplements, and it may then be shown to have some clinical success. Pycnogenol® has shown efficacy in patients with tinnitus and Meniere's syndrome and may be used on an individual basis in these subjects.

Andrology

Some andrological indications (decreased libido and erectile dysfunction) could be positively affected by DHEA and by a specific combination supplement (Prelox®). Prelox® is a combination of two ingredients, L-arginine and Pycnogenol®. It has been shown in several studies to increase blood flow and release vasospasm. The product is safe and well tolerated, and in a condition like erectile dysfunction which has so many hormonal, psychological and other components, Prelox® may have a significant role to play.

Other uses of PS supplements

Some concepts like "more energy" or "well-being" are very difficult to fit into a clinical context and are often meaningless. We do not discuss them in this text, as we are focusing predominantly upon clinical applications.

Athletic performance may be improved with CoQ10, creatine, DHEA, ginseng and with Pycnogenol®, but clinical situations are limited and out of the fields of interest for this text. It is likely that the most dubious supplements in this field are also outside the concept of sport. Specialists in *cocoonology* or *longevity* may have a different interest in prolonging life forever (see the paranoid media attention for resveratrol that basically has no evidence). Again, age is not a disease *per se* and Gerovital®-like supplements have probably passed their time, but they still have a market.

The use of some supplements for *cancers* (excluding some palliative applications) appears very difficult and controversial to manage, bordering criminal allegations. While there is (possibly) a correlation between the use of some supplements in the *daily diet* in some populations (e.g., curcumin) and the reduced incidence of some *cancers* (i.e., colon cancers, prostatic cancer), the logistical process required to transfer this information into clinical steps or using a supplement to decrease the frequency of cancers may require many years of man hours, thousands of patients and quite a lot of aggressive speculation.

In some cancer patients, side effects from radio- or chemotherapy are reduced by Pycnogenol® or curcumin administration (Meriva®), but this has nothing to do with the primary neoplastic disease, and we must be certain that the supplementary treatment does not interfere with the primary antineoplastic management. Therefore *cancers, cancer prevention and treatments* are not discussed in depth within this book as the evidence seems to be very weak and often confined to very basic cellular studies far away from clinical contexts. PS supplements and cancers are in different galaxies.

4

Testing PS Supplements: Organization of Supplement Studies

The 2013 London & Annecy panels

Clinical trials

Clinical trials are research studies that prospectively assign human participants or groups of humans to one or more health-related interventions to evaluate the effects on health outcomes. In an observational or registry study, without specific interventions, the investigators observe the subjects and measure their outcomes. The researchers do not actively manage the study.

Supplement studies

For supplement studies, the fields of activity, i.e., preclinical and borderline conditions or risk conditions, are clearly defined. Supplement studies produce comparative data or find presence of comparative, background, historical data for comparable subjects. Ideally, supplements help manage a risk condition of a pre-subclinical problem. Supplements are not used as drugs for a specific claim as treatment. Supplement studies suggest to patients or subjects the risk of supplement use (they do not prescribe) or supplement option. The patient or his/her caregiver will decide based on the suggestions.

Supplements are used in addition to the standard, best management/care for that condition. Supplements should not interfere with other treatments. The periods of follow up in the study may vary within a range and are not pre-fixed. The supplement should be administered as long as needed to see results or changes. Supplement studies aim to evaluate compliance in the use of supplements as a resulting critical factor. The methods of evaluation are as follows:

(a) retrospective analysis,
(b) noninterventional registry,
(c) observational study without specific interventions.

For these studies, there is no defined group allocation, no randomization, no placebo as these conditions necessarily lead to Good Clinical Practice (GCP) studies. *Open-label* patients always know what the supplementation, treatment and management are and what they can do. The net effect is the supplement action + a possible placebo action.

Any placebo effect is usually overconsidered and overevaluated. It should be positively managed in this type of evaluation. This conduct for supplement studies also much better resembles an actual preclinical or clinical use with all its implications. Most of the GCP studies are actually very artificial with defined age and sex definition and other characteristics that are rarely comparable with real, broad clinical use. Data are analyzed after a period of study when sufficient evidence is available or when it is possible; the analysis is postponed if funds are insufficient.

Characteristics of the study

Generally, supplement studies should be:

(a) small scale,
(b) independent,

(c) one-center studies,
(d) one in which the product (supplement) is not directly supplied,
(e) one that deals with the products that are generally available in the open market,
(f) one that guides patients get or buy the supplement product themselves.

The limited costs should allow anybody in the medical field to plan and organize these studies. Some studies could be organized by patients or consumers or subjects that have an interest in the problem. These studies could be very useful particularly in countries with limited budgets and when doctors and group of doctors have limited funds and resources and may be able to use the (locally produced) supplement instead of importing a more expensive product. Now GCP studies can only be organized by companies or important institutions with huge costs. Costly studies are only organized in view of anticipated high revenues.

Presence of external study reviewers: The definition of the role and activity of a possible, international *super partes* committee is in progress.

Advantages of supplement studies

The advantages of supplement studies are as follows:

(a) speed,
(b) low cost,
(c) availability for small centers, single physicians, low-budget institutions,
(d) possibility for local studies to evaluate local, natural products.

Exclusion: In the case of clinical problems and conditions, consider GCP studies.

When a supplement is intended to treat specific clinical conditions and a study is planned to have a claim, GCP studies should be planned, because it is not considered to be a supplement anymore. When looking for *defined claims*, GCP studies are needed, particularly when it is not possible to organize pilot, open-label studies.

Informed consent (IC)

Informed consent is now needed before any medical action, investigation, procedure or protocol. It is not specific for this kind of evaluation. For a supplement registry, you should not ask for another one, particularly if the patient decides to use the supplement by himself.

Notes on IC

Following are some notes on IC:

- The consent a person gives is based on understanding and all needed information must be given and discussed.
- IC is given only when based upon a clear understanding and acceptance of all the facts, implications and future consequences of a medical action.
- Most supplement administrations should follow only after the giving of IC. To give IC, the individual must have adequate reasoning faculties and be in possession of all relevant facts at the time consent is given.
- Impairment to reasoning/judgment makes IC impossible. Such situations may include basic intellectual or emotional immaturity, high stress (i.e., posttraumatic stress disorder) or severe mental deterioration or impairment, intoxication, severe sleep deprivation, Alzheimer's disease or coma.

Other points to expand

The 150 factor

Most PS supplements in their historical formats that have been tested and evaluated with a factor of 150/1 (subjects or patients) in comparison with "normal" patented prescription drugs are therefore, by definition, safer. PS supplements do not need prescriptions because they are considered safe and easy to use. This is not the case always, but it is an important assumption to be validated and verified for each supplement and for each application.

The one-shot, one-application factor for patented industrial prescription drugs makes them more "specialized" for specific applications and for selected groups of patients. Therefore, these products tend to be limited in experience and may be a source of problems if applied in a setting a that is not exactly corresponding to its specific, defined application (as seen in a clinical trial).

Animal studies and cell models

Animal studies are basically useless unless required to assess safety. Efficacy cannot be assessed with an animal model or cells, and the experience cannot be transferred to humans in any way. Diet, intestinal processing and absorption and metabolism of most complex supplements are completely different in different species. It is better not to mention animal models to confuse customers (i.e., cancer cells grow slower with some supplements). More than being useless, these statements can be dangerous and cause confusion and even determine or facilitate avoidance of "more proven" standard treatments.

Complex vs single molecules

Supplements are usually complex blends of molecules more than a single molecule (as most "patented" prescription drugs). It is their weakness as well as their strength. It is possible that within a complex supplement, some molecules may have a direct clinical effect and some other may facilitate either absorption or metabolism or the clinical effects or they may protect the healthy organs and cells from damage.

Terminology

In dealing with supplements, particularly PS supplements, there are some demeaning words to avoid, particularly when writing or speaking. It is important to limit confusion and to avoid degrading the potential reputation of the products.

Examples

Following are some examples of terms to be avoided to limit confusion and to avoid degrading the potential reputation of the products:

- *Phytotherapy* is something else, nothing to do with pharmaceutical formulations or PS supplements.
- *Alternative* is really misleading and gives most people and physicians bad feelings. These is nothing alternative in most PS supplements or in their applications. It is simply medicine.
- *Natural* is also another word to avoid. Natural has nothing to do with PS supplements that have been produced with a complex and often costly process including standardization.
- *Traditional* also sounds really bad.
- *Popular* is also to be avoided. It does not mean anything. Most of the PS supplements now available have important *historical* (rather than "traditional") roots, but minimal traditional ties, and are derived from a contemporary, complex and long pharmaceutical and industrial evolution.
- *Well-being* — a really abused term — does not mean anything from a physiological or clinical point of view. Any claim of "inducing well-being" should be dismissed with derision and viewed with suspicion. Well-being, if indeed there is anything at all with this name in medicine, is also a very personal concept. It cannot be reached with supplements or drugs, at least it should not. Anytime somebody mentions "well-being", there is something fishy/wrong, and it sounds shamanic, really bad from a scientific or clinical point of view.
- *Longevity* also is a confusing, misleading and abused concept. You cannot increase individual longevity as nobody knows the number of years you may have. It could be only a very generic, population concept. Making telomeres longer in worms or rats does not add very much to our life. There is not a single drug or supplement that can claim to change longevity.

In summary, language and culture changes *should be* significant tools to develop a new system to promote and market PS supplements. However, it is essential they should be linked to real physiological concepts, and to the medical field, with all its aspects and basic rules, including the important pharmaceutical process that produces them.

PS supplements, by definition, are intrinsically safe; they do not need prescription. It is impossible to kill yourself with a PS supplement or be killed, by mistake, by supplements. Phytotherapy, on the contrary, may kill. In the US alone, some 15 subjects a year are actually killed by more dangerous phytoproducts (e.g., ephedra, a medicinal preparation from the plant *Ephedra sinica*) used for weight loss. Concerns regarding the safety of ephedra supplements led the FDA to ban the sale of ephedra-containing supplements in the US in 2004. This ban was challenged by supplement manufacturers but was eventually maintained.

A review of ephedra-related adverse reactions, published in the *New England Journal of Medicine* in 2000, found a number of cases of sudden cardiac death or severe disability resulting from ephedra use, many of which occurred in young adults using ephedra in the labeled dosages. Therefore, all PS supplements should be safe and should not put the patient in any form of acute risk.

Supplements are often effective *on an individual basis* (this is very important in the age of individualized medicine), and they are a defined individual choice (supplements are not usually provided by healthcare systems) to buy personally at significant cost. A choice that costs is always an important choice to respect. PS supplements should obtain (with the same produce) the same consistent effects, time after time. Patients have the full opportunity to evaluate by themselves the possible positive effects and choose to use it or to stop supplementation.

Who is your customer?

Communications to physicians and pharmacists is the key form of promotion for many producers of PS supplements. *However, the real customer for supplements is the user, the patient that buys the product.* Physicians and pharmacists are just facilitators. The most important level of attention for producers of supplements should be toward their actual customers who buy the product expecting an effect and who deserve the complete attention and frankness of the producer.

General precautions: The US Food and Drug Administration (FDA) recommends to consumers that they inform their healthcare providers about supplements they may be taking, as some supplements may not be completely risk free under certain circumstances (i.e., use of other products) or may interact with prescription and over-the-counter medicines.

In conclusion, ideally a PS supplement should not cause problems even with accidental overdoses and should not kill any patient; it should be able to be declared safe and usable without prescription. There is a significant possibility that *combination products* have considerable applications at the moment, and in the future, there is little doubt that combination products will be able to be studied and developed. Many PS supplements already now include more than one product. The trend is increasing. The safety of each product should not be compromised by the combined use with another product, even if both products are safe. But safety, tolerability and potential interaction studies are still needed as the first step for each new combination, even before efficacy studies.

New evaluations in progress

Most supplements are combinations of several compounds. The cocktails are mostly effective when they include the full combination of compounds. The use of solvents or other complex pharmaceutical methods to extract single, separate elements from the combinations may produce a nonnatural compound that is not in the list of supplements (as it may include remnants of solvent or other extracting fractions).

The product could be significantly different from the original complex and expose patients to potentially unknown effects. *The metabolic pool* is a developing concept including all aspects involving the interactions between the PS supplement and the metabolic pathways. The metabolic pool and pathways could be completely different among different animals, particularly for complex cocktails of products or substances, and make animal studies mostly irrelevant.

The interactions in the pool may happen at intestinal level (i.e., altering absorption, competing for absorption of significant nutritional or toxic elements), a direct interaction with organs in the venous bloodstream before a first-pass effect, an interaction of the complex or single elements after a first-pass effect with partial or complete metabolization of some of the components (altering the composition of the complex). Also, protein or cellular binding and transport, extraction of significant elements from the bloodstream and organs could happen. The metabolic pool model must finally consider the late, possible actions of some remnants either metabolized or unmetabolized and the possible accumulation in specific storage elements (i.e., fat).

The model of the single pharma molecule, generally acting on specific receptors (as proposed for most prescription drugs), with a defined, constant metabolism in standard conditions is not valid for most supplements due to their pharmacological complexity. The model of the single molecule, selective drug is generally associated with a greater specific — and very selective — activity and to a greater danger of important side effects. The therapeutic range between collateral damage and pharmacological effect is a significant characteristic of molecular drugs, not shared by supplement complexes (lower efficacy, less specific, minimal danger of side effects). For each supplement, a specific metabolic pool should be defined and evaluated in the next few years.

Evaluation of thrombogenicity and compatibility with anticoagulants or antiplatelet agents

Anticoagulants are used very often in a larger number of subjects (with three main indications: thrombosis/embolism, valvular or device anticoagulation, fibrillation and cardiac prevention). The number of subjects using oral anticoagulants is increasing and also the number of subjects undergoing heparin prophylaxis (low-molecular-weight heparins and new heparins/heparinoids) is increasing. It is imperative, in the next few years, to define the antithrombogenetic or prothrombogenic activity of most supplements with specific tests. Also, the number of subjects >50 using antiplatelet agents is becoming astronomical, and possible interactions with antiplatelet agents should be evaluated.

Preventing bleeding at every level (e.g., at retinal level in diabetics or in the brain) of unwanted clotting (e.g., causing stroke or myocardial infarction) may reduce a significant number of events and medical, personal and social costs. Therefore, the safety evaluation protocols for PS supplements should now include the thrombogenesis aspect as it is likely that a great number of subjects using anticoagulants may use supplements, often even without medical prescription or suggestion.

Interactions with other commonly used drugs (antihypertensive, cholesterol-lowering drugs, antidiabetic agents) should be evaluated. The general, individual safety and the absolute safety of supplements is broadly valid for subjects not using other drugs/products and without associated clinical conditions but cannot be defined or granted for patients using a mix of drugs; that is, subjects with kidney or liver impairment may have a different response to some PS supplements that should be considered by a clinician.

Many of our patients (>35% for age >55), even in absence of important symptoms, have to use, on the basis of prescriptions, an antiplatelet agent, an antihypertensive drug and a lipid-lowering agent. Therefore, a healthy subject may buy a supplement and use it without problems of safety, but patients should always talk with their clinician and ask whether the use of the supplement is appropriate.

The safety factor: the safety table

Tolerability and safety should be the first concern for any PS supplement. Any study should include — as a preliminary step — the safety evaluation. Table 1 (including the seven pillars of safety) can be used as a reference.[1]

The historical use of most products for ages is a significant and clinically important historical evaluation. In centuries of use, any possible side effect or intolerance has not only emerged and been noted but has also been observed and confirmed several times. Most if not all side effects have been observed and reported and are generally incorporated into the historical profile of the product or extract in its different forms even when the product has not been used as a real PS supplement. The different side effects and tolerability stories of different extracts and formats are also generally known. Not a single "patented" drug usually used for a specific, single defined use or for a limited range of clinical applications could have the safety profile of any of these historical products.

Generally, the safety/tolerability profile of any of the historical popular supplements, even those not in a PS format, could be at least

[1] Belcaro, G. (2016). *Pharma-Standard Supplements*. Imperial College Press, London.

Table 1: The tolerability/safety scale: the seven pillars of tolerability.

			Scale score			
No.	Safety factor items	Range	0	1	2	3
1	Tolerability	0–3	Very good	Minimal	Significant	Severe
2	Doses assumed	0–3	100%	95–99%	75–94%	<75%
3	Side effects	0–3	None	Minimal	Significant	Severe
4	Suspension of treatment	0–3	No	One dose	More than five doses	Block
5	Treatment: subjectively unpleasant	0–3	No	Minimal	Significant	Severe
6	Need for medical attention	0–3	No	Minimal (discussion)	Prescription treatment	Hospital admission
7	Would continue supplementation?	0–3	Yes	If advised	Only if needed	No

Notes: If the total is <1, the tolerability/safety is considered optimal. If the total is >5 and <10, the tolerability/safety is not good and requires a specific safety study. In case of score >7, supplementation should be questioned and standards, dosages and need for supplementation should be reconsidered and suspended until full documentation is available.

some 150 times more validated, stronger and wider than any modern patented drug. These patented drugs, tested in a relatively small number of subjects (for short periods of time) in very standard conditions, have not been exposed to all the possible human, clinical, genetic, interactive combinations and backgrounds that may originate safety or tolerability problems. Most of the historical products, when found effective in managing one problem, have also been empirically used for similar clinical problems and conditions expanding the experience of these historical products and their safety/tolerability profile.

No patented drug has been tested for so long and widely and for so many conditions. Modern drugs last so long as their patent and are in the market at the most for a few decades without any possibility of acquiring this sort of profile. They may be dismissed before they can cause a rare complication. The only possible exception is aspirin or acetylsalicylic acid (ASA) that has a very wide range of applications and a long-standing, historical and popular background. *Of course, these clinical, simple evaluation steps (the seven pillars) should always be associated with a complete laboratory evaluation according to need and to specific target organs for each supplement.*

5

Conclusion

The world of supplements needs a change and a defined organization with new rules. At the moment, it is a mix of good (very few) and bad products, and good and bad information, followed by a lack of clear governance. Specific journals and meetings should define clinical aspects for each supplement. The clinical view is the key. Supplements can only be effectively used by professionals with a strong clinical background.

The evidence for a supplement's activity should have specific rules. Most of the clinical journals at the moment that claim evidence for industrial "patented" drugs are heavily sponsored by the drug industry. Pharmaceutical companies will spend millions on patented products that will offer even minimal benefit, possibly very marginal and not too different from valerian or other extracts or supplements that cannot be protected by a patent. The PS supplement world is basically excluded or badly tolerated and needs new stages.

The evolution of PS supplements may also consider the production of low-cost (not patented) products in low-income countries to be used, when and if possible, as possible alternatives to "patented", more expensive, important drugs. In medicine, evidence is only found when and if there is a very important commercial advantage. The industry of PS supplements generally defines a limited, small, not high-profit market — with limited patenting possibility — and cannot produce expensive research and therefore strong evidence.

Part 3
Final Comments

Concluding Comments

Complementary and alternative (if there is alternative) medicine (CAM) is a very difficult galaxy with many options, mostly unproven. They are always a golden opportunity for charlatans. The best experiment of blending Western-mainstream medicine and traditional (Chinese) elements of a significant social value was the medical system of the barefoot doctors (BDs) involving more than one billion subjects for a long period of time. Poverty is a great inspiration and a good sponsor.

Most CAM at the moment is the toy of New Ager, ex baby boomers. It promises to be different, transgressive, spiritual (in a world with little spirit). Meditation allows to look inside yourself, but it is not practised often. The world is outside. CAM looks "alternative", cool and different, with no connections with evil big pharmas. However, as seen in the BDs experiment, poverty is a stimulus much greater than boredom or coolness. Systems really find their ground when tested for needs. However, the value of many practices is a topic of discussion with friends. Meditation may show us in a different light; we may look more spiritual. Aspirin is less glamorous than yoga or acupunture, nothing to write home about. But after uncramping yourself from a Buddha position, you may find that a less glamorous nap on a sofa may give you more.

Most CAM adds some mystery. It may even add some sanctity (the instructor or "master" often behaves like Yoda), but you may suspect that a unity with a higher force is not so sure. *There is something in the CAM methods that may have medical value, but we need to find it, define it and be able to give a value to what we get. At the moment, in looking for this "something", the attitude is often wrong or speculative. Medicine needs to be effective and not cool.*

Quack medicine, charlatans are frequent in these domains bordering medicine. Television and web are "nets" to catch easy fish. However, not many studies are made on acupunture; there is no patent to exploit. Herbolariums are gold mines. Several institutions are exploring this field. Plants in their original status have minimal effect, often unpredictable, and the whole field needs evolution into standardizations toward pharmaceutical standards. *However, not many patents can be linked to natural products.*

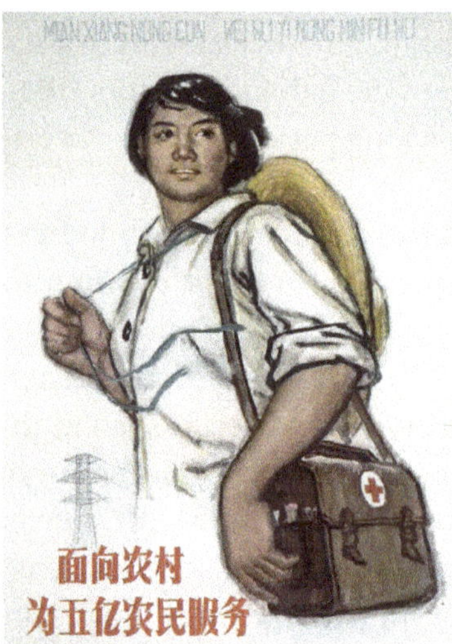

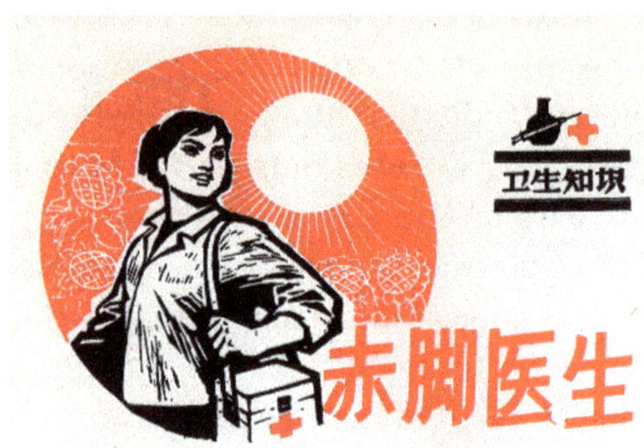

Dr. CAM meets Dr. Web

When considering CAM methods and system, we must now imply that the most important complementary–alternative system is the web. Patients continuously look for info, often for suggestions or directions, for diagnosis and mainly, eventually, for therapeutic solutions. The first CAM system is the web. It is the icebreaker and the lifeboat. Web evaluation is almost always uncritical, strongly self-promoting or market oriented and generally nonprofessional. Charlatans have found their stage. The present web is completely out of control.

Clinical cases used as anecdotal examples cannot scientifically compete with the evaluation of series in clinical studies. Most sites that sell drugs or supplements have no external or internal quality control. Web is expanding in its good and bad expressions mostly in dangerous directions. The low quality of web info — and products — induces a general low credibility on many medical systems that cannot compete in volume or quality. The diffusion of nonprescription products (no formal need for prescriptions) or the web sale of prescription products without prescriptions is a huge problem.

Directions and suggestions from a qualified professional are generally essential or at least very useful both to define activity and actions; but professional supervision also defines possible, important interactions with other "prescription" drugs. Qualified, nonprescription products should be recognized as safe (RAS) and ideally should not cause side effects. Still, a professional, medical guidance or supervision is essential. The most severe problem is the acquisition without prescription of drugs (prescription products) that may cause serious, even deadly, side effects and interactions.

Drugs are easily available in the web, at low cost and without formalities. One of the risks is that the actual drug is not present in the pill, and therefore there is no effect as expected. However, the dosages in the pill may be variable, not correct, excessive (rare), and some contaminant may be present in low-quality products. Some standard lipid-lowering drugs can be found in the web, in minutes, at prices some 10–20 times lower than the equivalent prescription product in the pharmacy. But the drugs are only the tip of the iceberg (and of the market).

Often, patients having a clinical problem — without professional advice or a formal diagnosis and clinical tests — are receiving treatment for another problem or just one symptom instead of a disease. The web is becoming a modern perimedical galaxy that sells more products than the regulated market, hosting an incredible number of gurus with obscure qualifications. The delay in obtaining a medical appointment, the increasing number of many, often useless expensive tests, considered essential for a diagnosis, bureaucracy, costs, the degraded contact with professionals and often the personal need to find a more adaptive diagnosis and treatment are all part of an equation forcing more and more subjects to accept the deformed web reality.

It is possible that the web may cause more clinical conditions than it may solve, complicating medicine that is becoming a mix of reality and unorthodox conceptions in a deadly confusion that may produce profits for many unqualified heath operators. In this unreal world, there is a lot of space for speculative CAMs that often rely on credulity more than science, on suggestions more than facts. It is a complex situation that is rapidly eroding the credibility and efficacy of the whole medical world and system. Physicians often have to face requests from deluded or confused patients who cannot easily discriminate navigation tips useful to avoid confusion. An explanation or an advice from a qualified website (i.e., the Mayo Clinic website) can be considered a good source of information, but some unqualified web advisers may mislead patients.

The trend now, particularly in the web, is an extension of "therapies" to normal subjects suggesting and marketing new "conditions" presented as a clinical problem (i.e., bloating, wellness, longevity) created just to sell some meaningless product or service. The dangers in using CAM methods is shown in Table 1. A *danger* score and a *safety* score are assigned to the most common methods. Figure 1 shows graphically the "danger" scores. Figure 2 shows a comparison of the danger and efficacy scores. Figure 3 shows the danger scores and safety profile. Table 2 shows the efficacy and safety scores (and a composite score). All these evaluations are arbitrary but involve a large number of subjects. Efficacy is based on how many patients (out of 10) find the method satisfactory on the basis of the symptoms (i.e., based on the CAM method used for producing a significant improvement or disappearance of the symptom in a comparable group of 10 patients).

The composite score is obtained by multiplying efficacy and safety scores (Figure 4). The composite score shows the relative value of each method. Below 20 (only two patients out of 10 have benefits), the method

Table 1: Dangers in using CAM methods (arbitrary danger score 0–10. 0 = no danger, 10 = it may kill).

Method	Danger score	Safety score
Naturopathy	10	0
Ayurveda	8	2
Homeopathy	7	3
Herbal treatment	7	3
Diet	5	5
Massage	3	7
Osteopathy	3	7
Yoga	3	7
Magnetotherapy	3	7
Chiropractic	2	8
Relaxation	2	8
Spiritual healing	2	8
Vitamins	2	8
Fields	1	9
PS supplements	0.5 (Nominal and RAS)	9.5

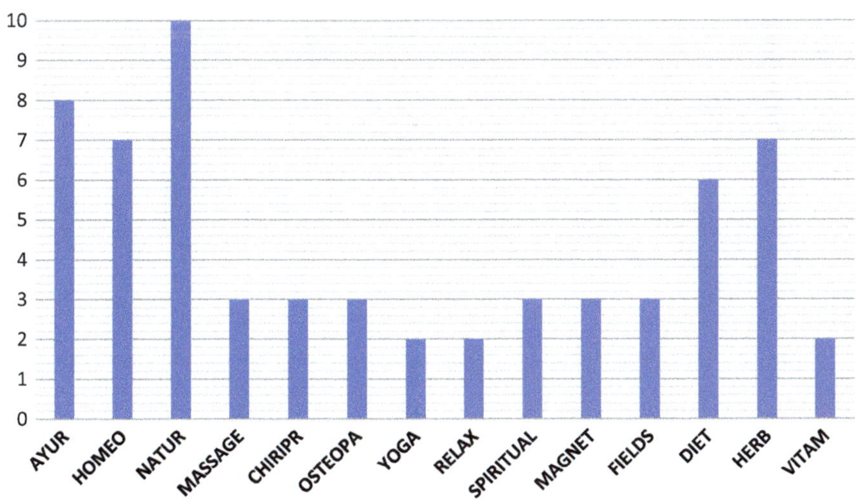

Figure 1: Danger scores.

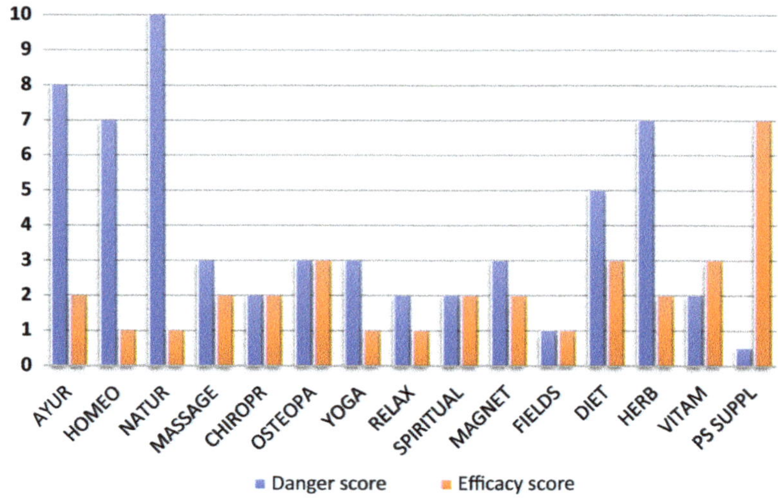

Figure 2: Danger score and efficacy score of CAM methods.

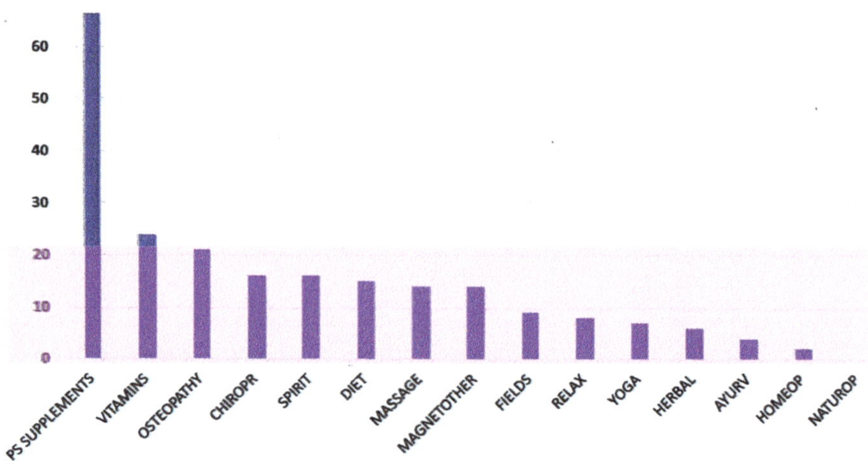

Figure 3: Danger score and safety profile for the most important CAM methods.

is basically useless. Most methods have no real standards, are very operator dependent and the diseases and signs/symptoms are often questionable.

Table 2: Efficacy and safety scores (and a composite score).

Method	Efficacy	Safety	Composite
PS supplements	7	9.5	66.5
Vitamins	3	8	24
Osteopathy	3	7	21
Diet	3	5	15
Ayurveda	2	2	4
Massage	2	7	14
Chiropractic	2	8	16
Spiritual healing	2	8	16
Herbal treatment	2	3	6
Magnetotherapy	2	7	14
Homeopathy	1	3	2
Yoga	1	7	7
Relaxation	1	8	8
Naturopathy	1	0	0
Fields	1	9	9

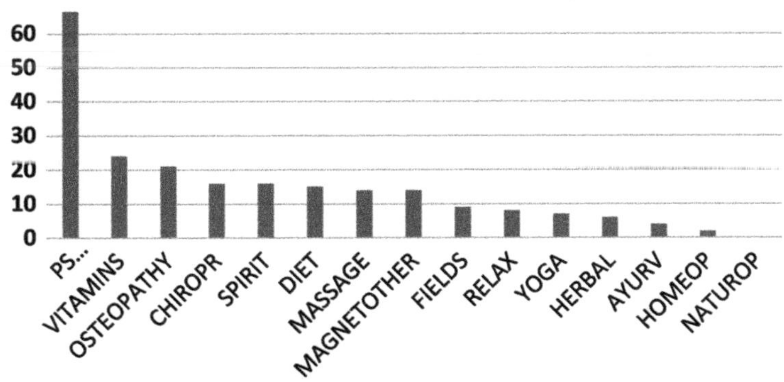

Figure 4: Composite CAM scores (safety scores multiplied by efficacy scores).

If we use a score 1–10 for the dangers present in a CAM method or system and an equivalent score for efficacy (1–10), it is possible to classify CAM methods from the most dangerous to the safest and from the less effective method to the most effective. Efficacy can be evaluated — and arbitrarily scored — by the patients or externally from a professional.

PS supplements — as expected — score the best in this pack due to their very high safety (products are recognized as safe) and their higher "clinical" efficacy; PS supplements have a significantly higher score in comparison with all other methods. However single, individual ("individual", meaning both the operator and the patient) responses may be considered and some methods may be used in selected patients in specific conditions or when no other management is possible or accepted. Ideally, all these methods should be always used in association with the best available, standard management.

Thermalism is considered in mainstream medicine, but it would score less than 20 in the composite score, and most physiotherapy methods would also have a very low score. If we also evaluate some mainstream medical methods, they would score below 20. There is no fluid or mysterious energy in hands. But we keep looking for it.

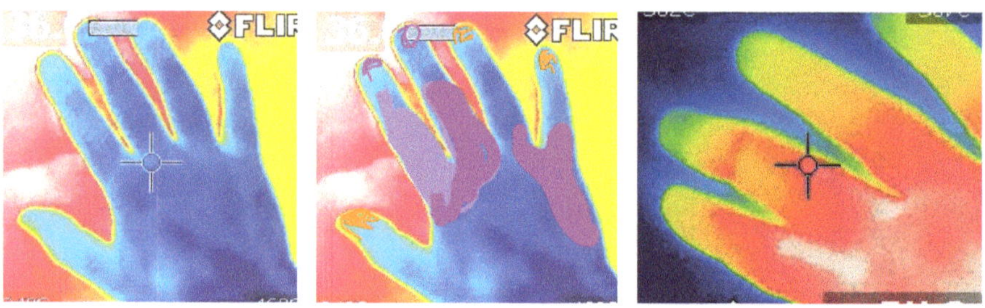

Thermal images of the hand.

Two misleading concepts without substance: holistic and integrative — words, just words

Holistic medicine

Holistic medicine (HM) — *a consideration of the complete person* (what "normal medicine" does) — *acts physically, psychologically, socially and spiritually in the management and prevention of disease.* The main concept of HM indicates that *there is a link between physical health and more general well-being*. This sentence does not mean anything, and well-being is not a medical or even physiological concept. The holistic approach to medicine considers that our *well-being* relies not only on what our body is physically in terms of illness/disease *but also on a close interrelation of body and psychological, emotional, social, spiritual and environmental status*. This is also what good, "normal medicine" does all the time. *These different states (spirit and so on) may be equally important and should be managed together so that a person is treated as a whole*. The concepts are misleading and try to convince, with a wording-based marketing strategy that "normal, mainstream medicine" does not consider these points.

Integrative medicine

Integrative medicine (IM) is apparently based on the definition of health by the World Health Organization (WHO) that defines health as "a state of complete physical, mental and social well-being and not merely the absence of disease or infirmity". So if there is no social well-being because there are social differences in class and income, the WHO should promote revolutions.

IM had the aim to restore and maintain health and *wellness* (again) *by understanding the patient's unique conditions and addressing all physical, emotional, mental, social, spiritual and environmental influences affecting health*. Same as before, this has no meaning. *Through personalizing care* (as standard medicine does), *IM goes beyond the management of symptoms to address all the causes of an illness* (mainstream medicine does exactly the same). IM, according to their Gurus, *responds to the patient's immediate health needs in association with the consideration of the long-term and complex interplay between biological, behavioral, psychosocial and environmental influences*. Again, this has no real meaning and is no different from what "normal medicine" does; the elaborate wording corresponds to a precise marketing strategy without substance. IM, according to its Gurus, is not the same as alternative medicine (this set of managements is used in place of conventional therapies) or complementary medicine (this methodology refers to healing modalities that complement standard managements).

Defining principles of IM are as follows:

- *Patient and practitioner are partners in the healing process* (the difference in knowledge makes them unequal partners in knowledge, power and emotions).
- *All factors influencing health, wellness and disease are taken into consideration, including body, mind, spirit and community as in mainstream medicine, no difference.* No mention about poverty.
- *IM physicians use all healing sciences* (all healing sciences are medicine) *to facilitate the body's innate healing power.* However, some immunosuppressed patients do not have healing powers.
- *Natural, effective, minimally invasive interventions* (this is also what medicine does) are used when possible. *IM — considered by its gurus as good medicine — is based on good science.* But there is very little evidence from a scientific point of view that IM has any real meaning or more meaning of "normal, mainstream medicine".
- *IM physicians are inquiry driven and open to new paradigms.* This sounds messianic. What is a new paradigm?
- *Alongside the concept of treatment, the broader concepts of health promotion and the prevention of illness are paramount.* So, IM "doctors" want to treat even those without a problem, just in case.
- *The care is personalized to best address the individual's unique conditions, needs and circumstances* as in mainstream medicine.

In conclusion, the words "integrative" and "holistic" are advertising but cannot be used for medical methodologies; they trick the mind…big words, little substance. In the galaxy of complementary, alternative medicines, still looking for Dr. Goodbar, the "soft–safe" medicine based on PS supplements, is the most interesting, getting a better image and scientific background in modern, daily studies.

A combination of *Centella asiatica* (CA) and Pycnogenol® is used to block the progression of atherosclerosis; it seems to offer very good results (delayed progression) with a very high level of safety. There is not a single prescription drug with the same effects. Also, irregular plaques with irregular density — due to the collagen-modulating activities of CA — become denser and less prone to embolization or ruptures (Figure 5).

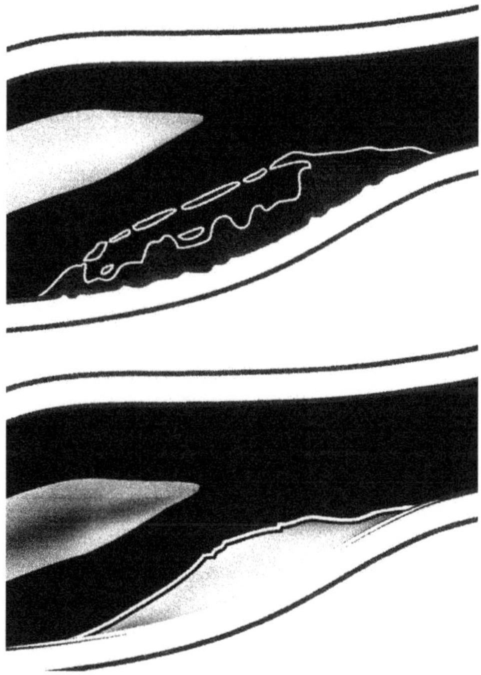

Figure 5: Carotid plaque with irregular components (top) becoming more dense and homogeneous (bottom) with management with *Centella asiatica*.

Final conclusion

This text is an expression of some starting points to base the research in this field (*complementary-supplementary medicine*) and will be followed by a much larger — more comprehensive — book in 3 y.[a]

[a] See *Pharma-Standard Supplements* by G. Belcaro (Imperial College Press).

Index

www.ingramcontent.com/pod-product-compliance
Ingram Content Group UK Ltd.
Pitfield, Milton Keynes, MK11 3LW, UK
UKHW022103170926
8624IPUK00024B/35

9 781786 345660